SUICIDE

SUICIDE

Edited by

Alec Roy, M.B., B. Chir.

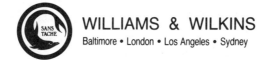

WILLIAMS & WILKINS
Baltimore • London • Los Angeles • Sydney

Editor: Nancy McSherry-Collins
Associate Editor: Victoria M. Vaughn
Copy Editor: Deborah K. Tourtlotte
Design: Bob Och
Illustration Planning: Lorraine Wrzosek
Production: Raymond E. Reter

Copyright © 1986
Williams & Wilkins
428 East Preston Street
Baltimore, MD 21202, U.S.A.

Printed in the United States of America

Library of Congress Cataloging-in-Publication Data

Suicide.

   Bibliography: p.
   Includes index.
   1. Suicide—Addresses, essays, lectures, I. Roy, Alec.
RC569.S92 1986   616.85'8445   85-20211
ISBN 0-683-07395-8

Composed and printed at the
Waverly Press, Inc.

86 87 88 89 90
10 9 8 7 6 5 4 3 2

For my parents,
Mary and George Roy

Preface

Suicide represents a major health problem. Between 0.5 and 1% of all deaths are due to suicide. We know from the classic studies of Robins and Murphy et al and Barraclough and Sainsbury et al that the great majority of suicide victims communicate their suicidal intentions and see physicians in the period before they commit suicide. Therefore, most suicides are probably preventable. Of all professional groups, psychiatrists have the most important part to play in suicide prevention. This is not only through their work in assessing and treating suicidal patients, but also through their important educational role. Psychiatrists in medical schools teach future physicians, psychiatrists in psychiatric hospitals teach future psychiatrists and psychiatric nurses, and in the community psychiatrists teach general practitioners.

The purpose of this book is to be a resource for psychiatrists and other mental health professionals. It is hoped that the psychiatrist in training faced with a difficult suicidal patient, or the psychiatrist with a lecture to give on suicide, will turn to this book and find it useful. As well as general chapters on definition, epidemiology, genetics, biochemistry, and management, there are chapters on suicide in relation to the major psychiatric disorders and to physical disorders. Suicide in adolescents is discussed in a separate chapter. Many of the leading suicide researchers kindly agreed to contribute to this volume, and in this fortunate circumstance some overlap has been accepted. Thanks are due to all of the contributors for their splendidly informative chapters.

Contributors

Marie Åsberg, M.D.
Professor of Psychiatry
Karolinska Institute
Stockholm, Sweden

Keith Hawton, D.M., M.R.C.Psych.
Consultant Psychiatrist
Warnefold Hospital
Clinical Lecturer in Psychiatry
University of Oxford
Oxford, England

Seymour S. Kety, M.D.
Professor Emeritus of Neuroscience
   in Psychiatry
Harvard University
Cambridge, Massachusetts
Associate Director for Basic Research
National Institute of Mental Health
Bethesda, Maryland

Norman Kreitman, M.D., F.R.C.P., F.R.C.Psych.
Director, Medical Research Council
   Unit of Epidemiological Studies in Psychiatry
Edinburgh, Scotland

George E. Murphy, M.D.
Professor of Psychiatry
Washington University School of Medicine
St. Louis, Missouri

Peter Nordström, M.D.
Department of Psychiatry
Karolinska Institute
Stockholm, Sweden

Eli Robins, M.D.
Professor of Psychiatry
Washington University School of Medicine
St. Louis, Missouri

Alec Roy, M.B., B.Chir., M.R.C.P., M.R.C.Psych.
Visiting Associate
National Institute of Mental Health
Bethesda, Maryland

Peter Sainsbury, M.D., F.R.C.P., F.R.C.Psych.
Lately Director of the Medical Research Council's
  Clinical Psychiatry Unit
Graylingwell Hospital
Chichester, Sussex, England

Phillip Seager, M.D., F.R.C.Psych.
Professor of Psychiatry
University of Shiffield
England

Edwin S. Shneidman, Ph.D.
Professor of Thanatology
University of California at Los Angeles
Los Angeles, California

Lil Träskman-Bendz, M.D.
Associate Professor of Psychiatry
Karolinska Institute
Stockholm, Sweden

F. A. Whitlock, M.D., F.R.C.P., F.R.C.Psych.
Emeritus Professor of Psychiatry
University of Queensland
Australia

Contents

1

Some Essentials of Suicide and Some Implications for Response

Edwin S. Shneidman, Ph.D.

The driving idea behind this chapter is the common-sense belief that effective therapy depends on assessment which is accurate and that accurate assessment depends on meaningful definition. Prevention rests on assessment; assessment rests on definition. When definitions are inadequate—"schizophrenia" as the towering example in the mental health field—it is unlikely that effective remediations can be found. The focus of concern is suicide, specifically suicide prevention.

We are coming up on the centennial of Durkheim's *Le Suicide* (1) and the 75th anniversary of the 1910 psychoanalytic pronuncimentos about self-destruction, and there is a feeling in the suicidological air that "the time is ripe" for some thoroughgoing reconsiderations of the nature of suicide, including, of course, the very definition of suicide itself. In this ambitious sense, these thoughts concern "the future of suicide," that is, how, in the immediate years to come, acts of suicide should be understood and how regarded, especially by the academic and professional communities.

In 1930 Maurice Halbwachs, a student and critic of Durkheim, set out to bring "up to date the work of Durkheim," but as he immersed himself further and further in his own data Halbwachs felt himself, to quote from the Foreward to *Les Causes du Suicide* (2), ". . . forced little by little to undertake new research, to pose new problems, to present the facts under a new aspect. In effect a totally new book was necessary."

But the sad fact is that Halbwachs' book on suicide was not at all a new approach. To quote from a contemporary of his: "The greatest part of Halbwachs' new facts on suicide were of the type Durkheim had described and were essentially subsumed by the interpretation which Durkheim proposed."

The point is: Bold words do not a new theory make. Many a self-proclaimed iconoclast ends up a tamed hagiographer. This author takes this as a cautionary for himself and as a caveat for each reader.

No contemporary suicidologist can eschew the formulations of either Durkheim or of Freud and the psychoanalytic school. There would be no point to do so. Nevertheless, there is merit in studying suicide by wholly independent routes, not neglecting those giants simply for the sake of avoidance, but consciously trying to create useful formulations other than the traditionally sociological or psychoanalytic ones. That is the route this author shall try to find.

DEFINITION OF SUICIDE

The basic word "suicide" needs to be clarified at the outset. The kind of suicide that will be discussed—its definitions and its characteristics—is what is commonly called *committed* suicide. The author well dislikes the terms "attempted suicide," "parasuicide," "threatened suicide," "inimical behavior," and "subintentioned death." A new term is needed for self-inflicted sublethal acts.

The term "attempted suicide" should be reserved for those rare cases of lethal intention in which the individual, against all ordinary odds, fortuitously survives. An example would be a case in which an individual puts a loaded, functioning gun to his head and pulls the trigger and the gun does not fire, or a person who immolates herself and survives. These people are special in the study of suicide.

But now, let us turn to committed suicides and begin with a few words about definition.

An apparently simple, straightforward definition of suicide, taken from the 1973 edition of the *Encyclopaedia Britannica* (3) is: "Suicide is the human act of self-inflicted, self-intentioned cessation." But there is more to it than that. One might make a tour of 20th-century definitions of suicide, fudging just a little bit and beginning with Durkheim. Durkheim's definition in 1897:

> "We may then say conclusively: The term suicide is applied to all cases of death resulting directly or indirectly from a positive or negative act of the victim himself which he knows will produce this result. An attempt is an act thus defined but falling short of actual death."

An exigesis, parsing, and dissection of this definition took Douglas (4) (*The Social Meanings of Suicide*) almost 400 pages to accomplish. Others, including Halbwachs (2), Achille-Delmas (5), Deshaies (6), Baechler (7), and Maris (8), have all wrestled with the topic of the definition of suicide without anyone—to be straightforward—pinning the idea to the conceptual mat for long enough for a suicidological referee to call a clear fall. Anyone who is interested in 20th-century definitions of suicide can find a good discussion in Baechler's *Suicides* and an excellent discussion in Douglas's *The Social Meanings of Suicide*.

The topic of the definition of suicide will be referred to again later. It is central to any efforts at a comprehensive discussion of therapy and response.

CLASSIFICATIONS OF SUICIDE

In contemporary suicidology the best known classification is still that of Durkheim. Every student of sociology can recite the three kinds of suicide—altruistic, egoistic, and anomic—and if he has read the footnote on the last page of the chapter on anomic suicide, a fourth type, fatalistic. In 1967, Douglas, in his analysis of definitions of suicide, listed six fundamental dimensions of meanings in definitions of suicide. The key words are *initiation* (of the act); the *act* (that leads to death); the *willing* (of self-destruction); the *loss* (*of will*); the *motivation* (to be dead); and the *knowledge* (of the death potential of the act).

In 1968, there was printed in the *Bulletin of Suicidology* (9) the suggestion that all suicides could be classified as egotic, dyadic, or ageneratic—a classification that was hardly mentioned thereafter. Baechler, in his substantial and interesting 1975 tome, *Suicides*, suggests four kinds of suicidal acts: escapist, aggressive, oblative (i.e., obligatory), and ludic (referring to games and play).

Currently, under the joint sponsorship of the American Medical Association and the American Psychiatric Association, there is an ongoing questionnaire study of 110 physician deaths by suicide and 110 matched nonsuicidal physician deaths. One would hope that their extensive questionnaire—over 130 questions in a 58-page booklet—

would reflect the current state of the art. The key question in that book, on the last page, reads as follows:

"How do you classify this suicide?
1. Rational (to escape pain, etc)
2. Reaction (following loss)
3. Vengeful (to punish someone else)
4. Manipulative (to thwart others' plans)
5. Psychotic (to fulfill a delusion)
6. 'Accidental' (reconsidered too late)."

It is easy to see some holes in that one.

All of these classifications, taken singly or together, have either an arbitrary, esoteric, or *ad hoc* quality to them. They do not seem impressively definitive. The best known of them is of practically no use in the clinic, where the task is saving lives, where conceptualizations count. In several years at the Los Angeles Suicide Prevention Center, the author never heard his colleagues or the county coroner refer to a suicidal death as altruistic, egoistic, or anomic. True, none of them was trained as a sociologist, but people not trained as psychoanalysts often employ psychoanalytic language, sometimes quite effectively. None of the classifications of suicide has an urgent usefulness.

To be theoretically serious about suicide, the author believes it best not to concentrate on classification, to eschew an attempt at taxonomy because, to use an anachronistic example, Linnaeus' perfect arrangement of all of Darwin's creatures is not an appropriate goal for a contemporary suicidologist. It was like trying to impose a biological screen on a variety of existential events. This follows Henry Murray's teaching that a discipline can be no more scientific than its subject matter will allow. A suicidologist is essentially a personologist. The accuracies of other fields of science, like physics or chemistry, are not consistent with what is known today about the activities, conscious and unconscious, of the human mind. The human person is, of course, the legitimate subject matter. There is no point in achieving accuracy if one sacrifices relevance in that process. A clinical suicidologist is interested in that which is useful and makes sense, not in what has specious accuracy.

COMMON CHARACTERISTICS OF COMMITTED SUICIDE

What are the interesting, relevant dimensions, that is, what are the *common* features or characteristics of suicide that can be delineated from a common-sense point of view, especially enlightened by systems theory attitude? The indispensable reference is Miller's monumental book, *Living Systems* (10).

A few words about the word "common" may be helpful. Each suicide is an idiosyncratic event. In suicide, there are no universals, absolutes, "alls." The best that one can reasonably hope to discuss are the most frequent (common) characteristics that accrue to most suicides, and to make this discussion in as common-sense and ordinary (and thus catholic) language as possible.

Following are some salient characteristics—the ten commonalities (see Table 1.1)—of suicide.

1. The common *purpose* of suicide is to seek a *solution.*

First, suicide is not a random act. It is never done pointlessly or purposelessly. It is a way out of a problem, a dilemma, a bind, a challenge, a difficulty, a crisis, an

Table 1.1. The 10 Commonalities of Suicide

1. The common purpose of suicide is to seek a solution.
2. The common goal of suicide is cessation of consciousness.
3. The common stimulus in suicide is intolerable psychological pain.
4. The common stressor in suicide is frustrated psychological needs.
5. The common emotion in suicide is hopelessness-helplessness.
6. The common internal attitude in suicide is ambivalence.
7. The common cognitive state in suicide is constriction.
8. The common action in suicide is egression.
9. The common interpersonal act in suicide is communication of intention.
10. The common consistency in suicide is with lifelong coping patterns.

unbearable situation. It has an inexorable logic and impetus of its own. It is the answer—the only available answer—to a real puzzler: How to get out of this? What to do? Its purpose is to solve a problem, to seek a solution to a problem generating intense suffering.

The well known English novelist and essayist, John Fowles, early in his career, wrote a brilliant set of aphorisms called *Aristos*. The Greek word *aristos* means the best possible solution in a given situation. The half dozen or more individuals with whom the author has talked who, in one way or another, attempted suicide—by immolating, jumping, or shooting—and fortuitously survived have all said something like, "It was the only thing I could do. It was the best way out of that terrible situation. It was the answer to the problem I had to solve. I couldn't see any other way."

In this sense every suicide is an *aristos*; every suicide has as its purpose the seeking of a solution to the perceived problem. To understand what a suicide was about, one has to know the problem it was intended to solve.

Therefore, the author offers this definition of suicide: Currently, in the Western world, suicide is the conscious act of self-induced annihilation, best understood as a multidimensional malaise in a needful individual who defines an issue for which the act is perceived as the best solution.

In Dante's *Commedia* there are nine poetically described descending circles in the Inferno to the ultimate devilish pit. In the real hell of life, the levels of misery seem endless. Except perhaps in the Nazi extermination camps, something worse than one's present awful state can usually be imagined. And it is that "something worse" that is feared. That is the common fear: the more pain, more degradation, more tension, more shame, more guilt, more terror, greater hopelessness, more insanity, something far worse, like having to survive and face the next day. To the extent that suicide is an act to solve a problem, the common fear that drives it is the fear that the situation will deteriorate, become much worse, get out of hand, excerbate beyond the point of any control. Better dead than mad. We have heard from the past generation of youths (and from psychologists) of ultimate moments, peak experiences, total actualization, complete emotional states, but life is much more realistically understood in terms, not of superlatives, but of comparatives. What we fear is something worse than what we have. Oftentimes, persons literally on the ledge of committing suicide would be willing to live if things, life, were only just a little bit better, a just noticeable difference more tolerable. The common fear is that the Inferno is bottomless and that the line on internal suffering must be drawn *somewhere*. Every suicide makes this statement: This far and no further—even though he would have been willing to live on the brink.

2. The common *goal* of suicide is *cessation* of consciousness.

In a curious and paradoxical way, suicide is both a moving toward and a moving away from something; the something that it is moving toward, the common practical goal of suicide, is the stopping of the flow of consciousness. Suicide is best understood not so much in relation as a moving toward the idea of a reified Death, as it is in terms of the idea (in the mind of the chief protagonist) of "cessation," specifically when cessation—the complete stopping of one's consciousness of unendurable pain—is seen by the suffering individual as a solution, indeed the perfect solution, of life's painful and pressing problems. The moment that the idea of the possibility of stopping consciousness occurs to the anguished mind as the answer or the way out in the presence of unusual constriction and elevated perturbation and high lethality—the three essential ingredients of suicide—then the igniting spark has been added and the active suicidal scenario has begun.

3. The common *stimulus* (or information input) in suicide is intolerable psychological *pain*.

If cessation is what the suicidal person is moving toward, pain is what that person is seeking to escape. In any close analysis, suicide is best understood as a combined movement toward cessation and as a movement away from intolerable emotion, unendurable pain, unacceptable anguish. No one commits suicide out of joy; no suicide is born out of exaltation. The enemy to life is pain, and, when pain does not come from one's own soma, then the threateners of life are those who cause the pain. It is psychological pain of which we are speaking, metapain, the pain of feeling pain. The clinical rule is: Reduce the level of suffering, often just a little bit, and the individual will choose to live.

4. The common *stressor* in suicide is frustrated psychological *needs*.

Suicide is best understood not so much as an unreasonable act—every suicide seems logical to the person who commits it given that person's major premises, style of syllogizing, and constricted focus—as it is a reaction to frustrated psychological needs. A suicide is committed because of thwarted or unfulfilled needs. In a wider sense, the systems theorist Ludwig von Bertalanffy (11)—emphasizing that self-destruction is intimately connected with man's symbolic and psychological world—says:

> "The man who kills himself because his life or career or business has gone wrong, does not do so because of the fact that his biological existence and survival are threatened, but rather because of his quasi-needs, that is, his needs on the symbolic level are frustrated."

But this author believes that psychological needs are not quasi-needs, nor are they symbolic. Needs are the very color and texture of our inner life.

In order to understand suicide in this kind of context, a much broader question needs to be asked, which is the key: What purposes do most human acts in general intend to accomplish? The best nondetailed answer to that question is that, in general, human acts are intended to satisfy a variety of human *needs*. There is no compelling a priori reason why a typology (or classification or taxonomy) of suicidal acts might not *parallel* a classification of *general* human needs. Indeed, such a classification of needs exists. It can be found in Murray's *Explorations in Personality* (12). These needs—some 20 in number—include the need for abasement, achievement, affiliation, aggression, autonomy, counteraction, defendance, deference, dominance, exhibition, harmavoidance (including painavoidance), infavoidance (relating to humiliation), inviolacy, nuturance, order, play, rejection, sentience, sex, succorance and understanding. There, in Murray's list of human needs, is a ready-made, viable, useful taxonomy of suicidal behaviors.

Each need can be related to a specific (psychological) kind of suicidal act. In Murray's discussion of needs, he further refines their place in human psychology by distinctions between covert and overt needs, between focal and diffuse needs, proactive and reactive needs, random and focused activities.

In each case, the lethal suicide act represents an effort by an individual to resolve a (real or fancied or exaggerated) problem either through the medium of satisfying that particular need (which, by the nature of the act, leads to death) or, pushed by a strong overriding general need, to satisfy that particular need specifically by means of a suicidal solution.

Most suicides probably represent *combinations* of various needs, so that a particular case of suicide might properly be subsumed under two or even three different need categories. An example would be a person who commits suicide by means of Russian roulette (by firing a bullet through the head with a one-out-of-six chance of death), largely because of a scandal in which that person's honor and reputation were impugned. Such an act (incident, occurrence, or event) would seem to have at least two components: (*a*) the need to avoid criticism, humiliation, blame, together with the need somehow to vindicate oneself or, to put it in a word, *defendance*; and (*b*) because in this case the technique of committing suicide is too dramatic to be disregarded, the need, in these dire straits, to play with one's life, to gamble with fate, to take excessive risks, to leave life itself up to chance, or, to put it in a word, *play*. (I shall use the word ludic here instead of play simply becauce the topic is too lugubrious to use this word with the more frivolous connotations.) Thus in this case, we might label that death as a "defendance-ludic suicide."

There are many pointless deaths, but there is never a needless suicide. Address the frustrated needs and the suicide will not occur.

The mental pain of the suicidal person relates to the frustration or blocking of important psychological needs, that is, needs deemed to be important by that person. The therapist's function is to help the patient in relation to those thwarted needs. Even a little bit of improvement can save a life. Oftentimes just the possibility of a small amount of gain gives the perturbed individual enough hope and comfort to divert the suicidal course. In general, the goal of psychotherapy is to increase the patient's psychological comfort. One way to operationalize this task is to focus on the thwarted needs. Questions such as "What is going on?"; "Where do you hurt?"; and "What would you like to have happen?" can usefully be asked by a therapist helping a suicidal person.

The psyochotherapist can focus on feelings, especially such distressing feelings as guilt, shame, fear, anger, thwarted ambition, unrequited love, hopelessness, helplessness, loneliness. The key is to improve the external and internal situations a just noticeable difference. This can be accomplished through a variety of methods: ventilation, interpretation, instruction, behavior modification, and realistic manipulation in the world outside the consultation room. That last means to do things, involve significant others, and invoke agencies. All this implies—when working with a highly lethal person—a heightened level of interaction during the period of elevated lethality. The therapist needs to work diligently, always giving the suicidal person realistic transfusions of hope until the perturbation intensity subsides enough to reduce the lethality to a tolerable, life-permitting level.

5. The common *emotion* in suicide is *hopelessness-helplessness.*

At the beginning of life the common emotion is probably randomized general excitement. In the suicidal state it is a pervasive feeling of hopelessness-helplessness: There is nothing that I can do (except to commit suicide) and there is no one who can help me (with the pain that I am suffering). This formulation permits us somewhat gracefully to withdraw from the (sibling) rivalry among the various emotions, each with the proponents to assert that *it* is the central of them all. Historically—in the 20th century, that is—hostility was the eldest brother. Stekel said so at the 1910 meeting of the Psychoanalytic Society in Vienna; no one kills himself except as he has fantacized the death of another. And then, in a somewhat more ornate phrase: Suicide is essentially hostility directed toward the (ambivalently viewed) introjected love object. One would plunge a knife into one's chest in order to expunge or kill the introject within of the loved-hated father—what this author once called murder in the 180th degree.

But today suicidologists know that there are other deep basic emotions: shame, guilt, frustrated dependency. The early psychoanalytic formulations are seen as a brilliant hypothesis, more pyrotechnical than universal.

But underlying all of these—and others that might be mentioned—is that emotion of active, impotent ennui, the feeling of hopelessness, helplessness.

6. The common *internal attitude* in suicide is *ambivalence.*

One does not ordinarily think of Freud as a giant in the history of logic but, in a way, he made as enormous an impact in extending the understanding of our cognitive maneuvers as perhaps Bacon, Mill, and Russell. In a word, Western logic is Aristotelian. (The topic of Eastern logic—see Nakamura's *The Ways of Thinking of Eastern Peoples* (13)—does not occupy us here, that is one reason why this author has never discussed Japanese and other Eastern suicides.) Aristotle's logic is dichotomous; more accurately, it is binary. A term is either A or non-A. An inference is either true or false; a mood of the syllogism is either valid or invalid. Except when one is arguing with one's spouse, as Socrates with Zantippe, the life of the mind is supposed to be rather straightforward; black or white, you might say. And that is what most people believe.

Freud brought to attention a psychological truth that transcends the Aristotelian appearance of the neatness of logic. Something can be *both* A and non-A. We can both like and dislike the same person; we can both love and hate a parent, a spouse, or a child. It is an Aristotelian question to say, Make up your mind! The answer is that we are of two minds, at least. The prototypical suicidal state is one in which an individual cuts his throat and cries for help at the same time, and is genuine in both of these acts. This non-Aristotelian accommodation to the psychological realities of mental life is called ambivalence. It is the common internal attitude toward suicide: to feel that one has to do it and, simultaneously, to yearn (and even plan) for rescue and intervention.

The core ambivalence in suicide reflects the main conflicts: between survival and unbearable stress. In response to the hostile and unfeeling question that, if a person wants to kill himself why not let him? one can answer that, if that same person wants to live why not throw in one's energies on the side of life? It is better not to visualize this as a struggle between, say, two figurative angels, the angel of death and the angel of life. It makes more sense to discuss this all-too-human conflict in concrete and effective terms and to answer that question, why not let him? by asking the practical counterquestion: Why not reduce the level of his unbearable stress? In effect, why not be a good Samaritan and *do* some things, often quite simple, inexpensive things, like talking to people, making arrangements, contacting agencies, manipulating intransigent people in the suicidal person's behalf? What the suicidal person requires is only the efforts of a benignant person, a champion, an ombudsman, a Samaritan.

7. The common *cognitive state* in suicide is *constriction*.

The author does not believe that suicide is best understood as a psychosis, a neurosis, or a character disorder. It is much more accurately seen as a more or less transient psychological constriction of affect and intellect. Synonyms for constriction are a tunneling or focusing or narrowing of the range of options usually available to *that* individual's consciousness when the mind is not panicked into dichotomous thinking: either some specific (almost magical) total solution *or* cessation; all or nothing; *Caesar aut nihil* (to quote from Binswanger's famous case of Ellen West (14)). The range of choices has narrowed to two–not much of a range. The usual life-sustaining images of loved ones are not disregarded. Worse, they are not even within the range of what is in the mind. Boris Pasternak (*I Remember*) (15), writing of the suicidal deaths of several young poets, described life-threatening constriction in this way:

> "A man who decides to commit suicide puts a full stop to his being, he turns his back on his past, he declares himself to be bankrupt and his memories to be unreal. They can no longer help or save him, he has put himself beyond their reach. The continuity of his inner life is broken, and his personality is at an end. And perhaps what finally makes him kill himself is not the firmness of his resolve but the unbearable quality of his anguish which belongs to no one, of this suffering in the absence of the sufferer, of this waiting which is empty because life has stopped and no one can feel it."

One of the most dangerous aspects of a suicidal state (high lethality/high perturbation) is the presence of constriction. Any attempt at rescue or remediation has to deal almost from the first with the pathological constriction.

People are often critical, prejudiced, and unforgiving about suicide; they forget that for the victim it is (also) a narrow-minded decision. This fact, that suicide is committed by individuals who are in a special constricted condition, leads to the suggestion that no one should commit suicide while disturbed. It is not a thing to do while one is not in one's best mind. Never kill yourself when you are suicidal. It takes a mind capable of scanning a range of options greater than two to make a decision as important as taking one's life. Dichotomous slogans like "death before dishonor," "live free or die," or "give me liberty or give me death" all have some emotional appeal, but they are not sensible or wide ranged enough to be prescriptions for making it through life.

It is vital to counter the suicidal person's constriction of thought by attempting to widen the mental blinders and to increase the number of options, certainly beyond the two options of either having some magical resolution or being dead.

An example may be useful. A teenage college student, demure, rather elegant (and somewhat wealthy) was encouraged to come to see the author. She was single, pregnant, and suicidal, with a formed suicidal plan. Her challenge was that the author somehow, magically, had to arrange for her to be the way she was before she became pregnant, virginal, in fact, or she would have to commit suicide. Her being pregnant was such a mortal shame to her, combined with strong feelings of rage and guilt, that she simply could not "bear to live." At that moment suicide was the *only* alternative for her.

The author did several things. He took out a sheet of paper and, to begin to "widen her blinders," said "Now, let's see: You could have an abortion here locally." ("I couldn't do that.") (It is precisely "can'ts" and "won'ts" and "have to's" and "nevers" and "always" and "onlys" that are negotiated in psychotherapy.) "You could go away and have an abortion." ("I couldn't do that.") "You could bring the baby to term and keep the baby." ("I couldn't do that.") "You could have the baby and adopt it out." ("I couldn't do that.") "We could get in touch with the young man involved" ("I couldn't do that.") "We could involve the help of your patents." ("I couldn't do that.") "You can always commit suicide, but there is obviously no need to do that today." (No response.) "Now, let's look at this list and rank them in order of your preference, keeping in mind that none of them is perfect."

The very making of this list and the author's nonhortatory and nonjudgmental approach already had a calming influence on her. Within a few minutes her lethality had begun to de-escalate. She actually rank ordered the list, commenting negatively on each item. What was of critical importance was that suicide was now no longer ranked first or second. We were then simply "haggling" about life—a perfectly viable solution.

The point is not how the issue was eventually resolved or what interpretations were made as to why she permitted herself to become pregnant, other aspects of her relationships with men, etc. What is important is that it was possible to achieve the assignment of that day: to lower her lethality by reducing her perturbation by widening her range of "logical" and realistic options from only the choice between suicide and one other choice.

The "logic of suicide" is a fascinating and complicated topic (as though the other aspects of suicide were not equally so). In other writings, the author has attempted to explicate the logics of two authors, Cesare Pavese, the 20th-century Italian novelist who committed suicide at age 42, and the special styles of logic contained in Herman Melville's masterpiece *Moby Dick* (16), which can be read as centering around the topic of self-destruction.

In working with a suicidal person it may be vital not to "buy into" his major premise (because all of his suicidal solution flows from that), but one should not argue or dispute the premise directly. Still, the key lies in not accepting the person's suicidal syllogism, his premises, and his lethal conclusion.

The logic of the suicidal person often contains a semantic fallacy that centers around the concept or word "I." It is a confusion of identification specifically between the individual as he experiences himself (I_s) and the individual as he is experienced by others (I_o). If an individual feels that as a result of his committing suicide, "I will be cried over; I will be attended to," then he is in the maelstrom of this confusion, for the "I" that he is talking about will no longer exist to receive those experiences.

The author terms this catalogic because the logic itself is destructive. The best set of illustrations of the logic of suicide can be found in *Moby Dick*.

In addition it is important to keep in mind that there is a latent syllogism in every suicide. The therapist should know what it is (in its manifest form) and should gently but firmly reject it by every interpretation and comment that is made to the suicidal person. Just as one does not collude with a suicidal person in fact, one should not collude with a suicidal person in logic.

Of course one's notions of death and life, one's cosmology, one's philosophy of life, one's epistemology are relevant to suicide. The idea of death is an essential ingredient of suicide; indeed, it is the igniting spark. However, while there is some idea of life and death in the suicidal complex, the particular form that it takes does not seem much to matter.

Stephen Pepper, late Mills Professor of Intellectual and Moral Philosophy at the University of California, Berkeley, has provided the golden grid. In his indispensable book, *World Hypotheses* (17), he argues, totally convincingly to this reader, that all philosophies ever enunciated—Socrates, Plato, Aristotle, etc; Descartes, Spinoza, Hume, etc; Kant, Schopenhauer, Nietzsche, etc; Carnap, Wittenstein, Ayer, etc; Kierkegaard, Jaspers, Satre, etc; *all*—can be subsumed under six rubrics, which he calls root metaphors or world hypotheses.

They are *animistic* world hypotheses, in which man and spirit are the primary root metaphors; *mystical* world hypotheses in which mystical experiences are the root metaphors—Pepper considers these two inadequate hypotheses because of their imprecision or limited scope (and their potentialities for destructiveness)—and four adequate world hypotheses: *formism*, in which the root metaphor is similarity; *mechanism*, in which the root metaphor is a machine; *contextualism*, in which the root metaphor is the historical event; and *organicism*, in which the root metaphor is historical process, especially the integration appearing in the process.

Among all suicides, vocalized and silent beliefs are distributed in some empirically to be determined way among these six world hypotheses. And since none of the six is an inoculation against suicide, one might conclude that the specific root metaphor would seem to be irrelevant to suicide. Nevertheless, it remains true that *some* concept of naughtment, oblivionation, death, or cessation is a sine qua non for the initiation of the suicidal drama. Although any credal religion has some life-enhancing implications, it also, especially when combined with elevated perturbation and constriction (which the creed may exacerbate), may contain significant life-diminishing (and suicide-promoting) components. In the long run, credal beliefs may hasten more deaths than they save lives. Pepper concludes one of his articles, "Can a Philosophy Make One Philosophical?" (18), with these reflections:

> "The rational guidance of a philosophy of life is available ony to a relatively well-integrated personality whose unconscious conflicts (such as he has) do not overpower his voluntary actions. To such a man an adequate philosophy would be his safest guide through life. And to my mind, for all who are in a position to acquire it, an explicit philosophy is a guide greatly superior to a purely institutionalized ideology or creed. For even when not inadequate, the latter is rigid and dogmatic, whereas the former may be flexible and open to revision."

8. The common *action* in suicide is *escape* (egression).

Egression is a person's intended departure from a region of distress. Suicide is the ultimate egression, beside which running away from home, quitting a job, deserting an army, or leaving a spouse pales. Erving Goffman spoke of unpluggings: having a good read, darting into a movie, going for a weekend to Las Vegas or Atlantic City— benign egressions all. But it is necessary to distinguish between the wish to get away and the need to end it all, to stop it for real. The point of suicide is a radical and permanent change of scene, the action to effect it is to leave.

Here is an excerpt from a letter, dated March 26, 1921, from Violet Keppel Trefusis to her lover Vita Sackville-West, then in the eight year of her unusual bisexual marriage to Harold Nicolson (19):

> "I am dead with grief. I am utterly alone. You cannot want me to suffer so.
> You had to choose between me and your family, and you have chosen them.
> I do not blame you. But you must not blame me if one day I seek for what
> escape I can find."

In the only unnecessary line in that fascinating book, Nigel Nicolson explains that that passage refers to suicide. Indeed, it is an operational definition of what, at rock bottom, from the suicidal person's point of view, suicide is: "... escape I can find." In that brief quotation from the letter, one can see intimations of several common characteristics of suicide: the wish for cessation, the need to stop pain, the sense of hopelessness, the presence of constriction, and the search for escape, as well as the communication of the intent.

In a special discussion of Melville (20), Henry Murray discusses suicide and egression. Murray states that not only is suicide total egression but that egressions can be fractional, like partial suicides. He thus opens up to us the vast topic of what this author, stimulated by his thoughts, came to call subintentioned death. Here is a key paragraph from Murray:

> '... we can see that egression not only may be, as it is in many cases, the
> expedient substitute for total suicide (insofar as it results in a surcease of
> pain), but ultimately, in some rare cases, may constitute a willful, partial
> suicide by taking the egressor beyond the tolerance of his fellowmen and of
> his own conscience, or, in other words, to the point where he is as good as
> dead in the affections of the world and of the "personified impersonal," and
> *they* are as good as dead in *his* affections."

That kind of living death, social suicide, is a topic too large for the present discussion. Suffice it to say that the omnipresent feature of the act of suicide is egression; it is a death in which the decedant takes himself from others in the world.

9. The common *interpersonal act* in suicide is *communication of intention.*

Perhaps the most interesting finding from large numbers of retrospective psychological autopsies of unequivocal suicidal deaths is that in the vast majority there were clear clues to the impending lethal event. These clues to suicide are present in approximately 80% of suicidal deaths. Individuals intent on commiting suicide, albeit ambivalently minded about it, consciously or unconsciously emit signals of distress, whimpers of helplessness, pleas for response, and opportunities for rescue in the usually dyadic interplay that is an integral part of the suicidal drama. It is a sad and paradoxical thing to note that the common interpersonal act of suicide is not hostility, not rage or destruction, not even withdrawal, but communication of intention.

Suicidologists now know the usual clues, verbal and behavioral. The verbal statements are tantamount to saying, "I am going away (egression); you won't be seeing me; I cannot endure it (pain) any longer"; the behavioral signs are such unusual acts as the person's putting his affairs in order, giving away prized possessions, and generally behaving in ways that are different from his usual behaviors and that betoken a bubbling (as a cauldron bubbles) in a perturbed psyche.

The communication of suicidal intention is not always a cry for help. First, it is not always a cry; it can be a shout or a murmur or the loud communication of unspoken silences. And it is not always for help; it can be for autonomy or inviolacy or any of a number of other needs. Nonetheless, in most cases of suicide, the common penultimate act is some interpersonal communicative exchange related to that intended final act.

10. The common *consistency* in suicide is *with lifelong coping patterns*.

People who are dying over weeks or months of a disease, say cancer, are very much themselves, even exaggerations of their normal selves. Contrary to some currently popular notions, there does *not* seem to be any standard set of stages in the dying process through which individuals are marched, lock-step, to their deaths. In terms of emotions displayed (rage, acceptance, etc) or mechanisms of psychological defense manifested (projection, denial, etc) one sees a full panoply of both of these arranged in almost every conceivable number and order. What one does see in almost every case are certain consistencies of display of emotion and use of defense that are consistent with *that* individual's microtemporal, mesotemporal, and macrotemporal reactions to pain, threat, failure, powerlessness, and duress in previous episodes of that life. People dying are enormously consistent with themselves. So are suicidal people. So are people who are neither dying nor suicidal.

In suicide, we are initially thrown off the scent because suicide is an act, by definition, which that individual has never done before so there is no precedent. And yet there are some consistencies with lifelong coping patterns. We must look to previous episodes of disturbance, to capacity to endure psychological pain, to the penchant for constriction and dichotomous thinking, for earlier paradigms of egression.

The author speaks with some experimental authority on this issue, at least with a sense of conviction that flows from the data he examined. Very briefly, he studied a group of men who were about 55 years old, each of whom had been studied rather intensively on a continual basis since he was about 6 years old (the well known Terman longitudinal study of the gifted, which began in 1920 with 1528 young male and female subjects and continues to this date at Stanford University under the direction of Professor Robert Sears). In the author's small study, other than the demonstration that it was possible (beyond chance expectation) to select the five subjects who had committed suicide from a group of 30 cases, the main finding was that—working as he did, from a detailed life-chart constructed for each individual—the determination that the person would (or would not) commit suicide at around age 55 could be made by the author before the thirtieth birthday in each man's life. There were already certain psychological consistencies within the life, certain characteristics or habitual patterns of reaction for that person to threat, pain, pressure, and failure which made dire predictions of a tragic suicidal outcome at 55 an almost straightforward, logical (and perhaps psychological) extrapolation.

Who, reading the several adolescent entries in the diary of the great 20th-century Italian writer, Cesare Pavese, and his detailed notations in his twenties is truly surprised by his last entry—"Not words. An act. I'll write no more."—and at his suicide at age 42? In the sight of the enormous unpredictability of life, what impresses and excites this author as a psychologist is how much of a person's life, in some of its more important aspects, is reasonably predictable. In general, he feels this way about suicide. It is enormously complicated, but it is not totally random, and it is amenable to some prediction. That is the main handle on individual prevention.

REFLECTIONS ABOUT SUICIDE AND ITS PREVENTION
The *universal* psychodynamic *formulation* for suicide is nonexistent.

One does not regret that suicidology is a different discipline from physiology or physics. One simply notes that it is and reflects upon it—different subject matters, different relevant methodologies, and different degrees of ultimate veridicality. The possibilities for some prediction have been discussed but not prediction with the precision of the physiologist or physicist; the author does not aspire to that level and does not think it should be wished for. When one's subject matter is the mind, one can be no more accurate or scientific than the relevant ways of investigating the subject matter will currently permit.

And yet the yearning for universal suicidological laws understandably persists. A sweeping psychological statement with the ring of psychodynamic truth in it becomes a dictum. The author believes, and not sadly, that the search for a single universal psychodynamic formulation for suicide is a chimera, an imaginary and nonexistent conceptual monster. There should be no sense of loss in this: This view simply redefines who we are, what our legitimate business is, and what our sensible goals ought to be.

If there are common psychodynamics in suicide they probably relate to omnipotence and loss. In the unconscious every suicide is psychodynamically related, directly or indirectly, to feelings of omnipotence-impotence; to feelings of being all-powerful and powerless-helpless. Suicide is an effort to do *something*, to do something effective, impactful, dramatic, memorable, noteworthy, special. A suicide would not be a suicide if it were unknown as a suicide.

Being known as a suicide is an integral part of the act. If, for example, a person has an extramarital affair and then tells the spouse about it, there are then two events: the affair and the telling. In suicide these elements are combined; the act and the telling are one. (That is why, in a sense, suicide notes are poignant redundancies. They unnecessarily restate what is instantenously obvious to the survivor on sighting the dead body.)

Suicide, like all deaths, while occurring in a dyadic setting, is, at bottom, an egotic (individual, solo, private) act. It is a one-person deed relating to that person's conscious and unconscious concern with active mastery, which, at its furthermost remove, relates to omnipotence. At the moment of committing suicide, the individual may feel he controls the world and by his death can bring it down. At least he controls his own destiny, and realistically he typically touches and influences the destinies of at least several others.

The great loss in suicide is the loss of the self. The main psychological focus of every formed person is with himself or herself. One is endlessly taken with the processes of his own mind, even if he does not reflect upon them. One's greatest fealty and loyalty is to himself. (This is not identical to narcissism, as it is currently understood.) The great mourning of the suicidal person is premourning, the mourning for the potential loss of the best known and best loved person in the world, the self.

A handsome young man who was a homosexual prostitute by profession and who was dying of leukemia, said: "Now a perfectly good person is going to die and the world will be poorer for it." He spoke a universal truth.

The *immediate antidote* for suicide is *reduction of perturbation.*

Now one comes to "the good stuff," helping people in distress. Suicide is best understood not so much in terms of some sets of nosological boxes, e.g., depression or any of the often sterile labels in the American Psychiatric Association's *Diagnostic and Statistical Manual of Mental Disorders*, but rather in terms of two continua of general personality functioning: *perturbation* and *lethality.* Everyone is rateable (by oneself or others) on how disturbed or distressed or upset (perturbation) he is and, additionally, on how deathfully suicidal (lethality) he is.

To say that an individual is "disturbed" or "suicidal" simply indicates that there is an elevation in that individual's perturbation and lethality levels, respectively. Moreover, it often happens that an individual is highly perturbed but not suicidal. It infrequently occurs that an individual is highly lethal but not perturbed. Experience has taught the important fact that it is neither possible nor practical in an individual who is highly lethal and highly perturbed to attempt to deal with the lethality directly, either by moral suasion, confrontatory interpretations, exhortation, or whatever. (It does not work any better in suicide than it does in alcoholism.) The most effective way to reduce elevated lethality is by doing so indirectly, that is, by reducing the elevated perturbation. Reduce the person's anguish, tension, and pain and his level of lethality will concomitantly come down, for it is the elevated perturbation that drives and fuels the elevated lethality.

With a highly lethal suicidal person the main goal is, of course, to reduce the elevated lethality. The most important rule to follow is that *high lethality is reduced by reducing the person's sense of perturbation.* One way to do this is by addressing in a practical way those in-the-world things that can be changed if ever so slightly. In a sensible manner, the therapist should contact the patient's spouse, lover, employer, government agencies, etc. In these contacts the therapist acts as ombudsman for the patient, promoting his or her interests and welfare. The subgoal is to reduce the real-life pressures that are driving up the patient's sense of perturbation.

A psychotherapist decreases the elevated perturbation of a highly suicidal person by doing almost everything possible to cater to the infantile idiosyncrasies, the dependency needs, the sense of pressure and futility, and the feelings of hopelessness and helplessness that the individual is experiencing. In order to help a highly lethal person, one should involve others; create activity around the person; do what he or she wants done, and, if that cannot be accomplished, at least move in the direction of the desired goals to some substitute goals that approximate those which have been lost. Remind the patient that life is often the choice among undesirable alternatives. The key to well functioning is often to choose the least awful alternative that is practically attainable.

The basic principle is this: To decrease lethality one puts a hook on perturbation and, doing what needs to be done, pulls the level of perturbation down, and with that action brings down the active level of lethality. When the person is no longer highly suicidal the usual methods of psychotherapy can be usefully employed.

The *intermediate response* to suicide is *to increase awareness of other adjustment processes.*

The key to intermediate and long range effectiveness of help with a suicidal person is to increase the options for action and to increase the ways available within and to the person to have more options—in a phrase, to widen the blinders. The suicidal act is an effort to stop unbearable anguish or intolerable pain by the individual's "doing something." Knowing this usually guides one to what the treatment should be. In the same sense, the way to save a person's life is by doing something. These "somethings" include putting that information (that the person is in suicidal trouble) into certain streams of communication, letting others know about it, talking to the persons, proferring help, getting loved ones to respond, involving agencies and organizations, creating action around the person, showing response, and indicating concern.

The only way to come back from a suicidal abyss and to stay on relatively firm ground is to grow, specifically to become aware of adjustment processes previously not prominent in one's armamentarium of techniques. In this regard the author has a rather catholic view: he certainly embraces the Samaritans and the activities of suicide prevention centers; he endorses psychotherapy, counseling, outreach, groups, and agencies. He has become tolerant of behavior modification techniques and role modeling, living in a home that fosters love, living in a loving foster home—anything that increases the person's awareness of adjustment processes being those of choosing between perceived misery and ambivalently viewed awful escape.

A highly suicidal state is characterized by its transient quality, its pervasive ambivalence and its dyadic nature. Psychotherapists are well advised to minimize, if not totally to disregard, those probably well intentioned but shrill writings in this field which naively speak of an individual's "right to commit suicide," a right which in actuality cannot be denied.

Several other special features in the management of a highly lethal patient can be mentioned. Some of these special therapeutic strategms or orientations reflect the *transient, ambivalent,* and *dyadic* aspects of almost all suicide acts:

1. *Monitoring*: A continuous (preferably daily) monitoring of the patient's lethality.

2. *Consultation*: There is almost no instance in a psychotherapist's professional life when consultation with a peer is as important as when one is dealing with a highly suicidal patient.

3. *Transference*: The successful treatment of a highly suicidal person depends heavily on the transference. The therapist can be active, show his personal concern, increase the frequency of the sessions, invoke the magic of the unique therapist-patient relationship, be less of a tabula rasa, give transfusions of (realistic) hope and succorance. In a figurative sense Eros can work wonders against Thanatos.

4. *The involvement of significant others*: Suicide is often a highly charged dyadic crisis. It follows from this that the therapist, unlike his usual practice of dealing almost exclusively with his patient (and even fending off the spouse, lover, parents, and grown children) should consider the advisability of working directly with the significant others. If the individual is married, it is important to meet the spouse. The therapist must assess whether, in fact, the spouse is suicidogenic; whether they ought to be separated; whether there are misunderstandings which the therapist can help to resolve; or to what extent that person is insightful and concerned. At the minimum the spouse's role as hinderer or helper in the treatment process needs to be assessed.

5. *Careful considerations of the usual canons of confidentiality*: Admittedly this is a touchy and complicated point, but the therapist should not ally himself with death. Statements given during the therapy session relating to the patient's overt suicidal (or homicidal) plans should not be treated as a secret between two collusive partners.

Working with highly suicidal persons borrows from the goals of befriending and crisis intervention: not to take on and attempt to ameliorate the individual's entire personality structure and cure all the neuroses but simply to keep the person alive. This is the sine qua non without which all other psychotherapy and efforts to be helpful could not have the opportunity to function.

The *ultimate prevention* of suicide is *public education* about the clues to suicide.

Most people would agree that the best prevention is primary prevention; an ounce of prevention is worth a pound of cure. The primary prevention of suicide lies in education. The route is through teaching one another and that large, amorphous group known as the public that suicide can happen to anyone, that there are clues that can be looked for (if one but has the threshold to see and hear them when they occur), and that help is available. Perhaps our main task lies in the dissemination of information, especially about the clues to suicide: in the schools, in the workplace, through the public media. In the end, effective prevention of suicide is everybody's business.

References

1. Durkheim E: *Suicide.* Glencoe, IL, The Free Press, 1951. (Originally published as *Le Suicide,* 1897.)
2. Halbwachs M: *Les Causes du Suicide.* Paris, Felix Alcan, 1930.
3. Shneidman ES: Suicide. *Encyclopaedia Britannica.* Chicago, William Benton, 1973.
4. Douglas JD: *The Social Meanings of Suicide.* Princeton, Princeton University Press, 1967.
5. Achille-Delmas F: *Psychopathologie du Suicide.* Paris, Felix Alcan, 1932.
6. Deshaies G: *Psychologie du Suicide.* Paris, Presses Universitaires de France, 1947.
7. Baechler J: *Suicides.* New York, Basic Books, 1979. (Originally published as *Les Suicides,* 1975.)
8. Maris R: *Pathways to Suicide.* Baltimore, Johns Hopkins University Press, 1981.
9. Shneidman ES: Classifications of suicidal phenomena. *Bull Suicidol* 1:1–9, 1968.
10. Miller James Grier. *Living Systems.* New York: McGraw-Hill, 1978.
11. von Bertalanffy L: *General Systems Theory.* New York, G Braziller, 1968.
12. Murray HA: *Explorations in Personality.* New York, Oxford University Press, 1938.
13. Nakamura H: *The Ways of Thinking of Eastern Peoples.* New York, UNESCO, 1967.
14. Binswanger L: The case of Ellen West. In May R, et al (eds): *Existence.* New York, Basic Books, 1958.
15. Pasternak B: *I Remember: Sketch for an Autobiography.* New York, Pantheon, 1959.
16. Melville, H: *Moby Dick.* New York, New American Library, 1985.
17. Pepper SC: *World Hypotheses.* Berkeley, University of California Press, 1942.
18. Pepper SC: Can a philosophy make one philosophical? In Shneidman ES (ed): *Essays in Self-Destruction.* New York, Science House, 1967.
19. Nicolson N: *Portrait of a Marriage.* New York, Atheneum, 1973.
20. Murray HA: Dead to the world. In Shneidman ES (ed): *Essays in Self-Destruction.* New York, Science House, 1967.

2

The Epidemiology of Suicide

Peter Sainsbury, M.D., F.R.C.P., F.R.C. Psych.

Of all the deviant forms of human behavior, suicide is probably the one most suited to epidemiological research. The reasons for this are that the epidemiologist's two major problems of method—defining the case and finding all the cases in the population—are largely taken care of by the statutory procedures for investigating violent or unexpected deaths (a claim that will be considered more fully below). In addition, abundant mortality statistics are available, in some countries extending for over a century, so that the rates of different social and demographic groups may be compared, trends studied, and the ecology of suicide explored. Moreover, the epidemiological method can be amplified by combining it with the case-study approach in which selected features of consecutive suicides and matched controls from a population are compared (1).

The purpose of this chapter, therefore, is to examine factors which affect the frequency and distribution of suicide. This will entail considering the extent of the problem and then identifying those social and demographic groups most at risk in order to devise ways of preventing suicide, on the one hand, and to explore social and other circumstances that predispose to it, on the other.

The wealth of epidemiological information on suicide not only provides data from which to test hypotheses about factors predisposing to it, but also to certain psychiatric disorders, since evidence indicates that nearly all suicides have an overt mental illness (see Chapter 9).

THE ACCURACY OF SUICIDE STATISTICS

The principal sources of data on suicide are the official mortality statistics which most countries publish. However, the accuracy and comparability of suicide rates so derived, hence their value for purposes of epidemiological research, have been questioned (2, 3).

First, critics argue that the differences in national rates of suicide are invalid because countries differ in their procedures for ascertaining and reporting suicide. In order to investigate this claim, Sainsbury and Barraclough (4) compared the suicide rates of immigrants to the United States from 11 countries and found that their rates rank in the same order as do the suicide rates of their countries of origin (see Table 2.1).

Since suicide is ascertained in the US by procedures particular to that country, whereas different procedures obtain in each of the countries from which emigration occurred, it follows that the differences between the nations' suicide rates cannot be due to variations in the ascertainment of suicide, so other sociocultural consideration must be invoked to account for divergences in national rates. This conclusion was

Table 2.1. Suicide Rates per 100,000 Immigrants to the United States for 11 Countries, 1959*

Country	A Suicide rate/ 100,000 of Foreign Born in US (1959)	B Suicide rate/ 100,000 of Country of Origin (1959)	Rank Order of A	Rank Order of B
Sweden	34.2	18.1	1	4
Austria	32.5	24.8	2	2
Czechoslovakia	31.5	24.9	3	1
Germany, Federal Republic	25.7	18.7	4	3
Poland	25.2	8.0	5	6
Norway	23.7	7.8	6	7
England and Wales	19.2	11.5	7	5
Italy	18.2	6.2	8	9
Canada	17.5	7.4	9	8
Ireland	9.8	2.5	10	10
Mexico	7.9	2.1	11	11
United States	10.4			

$rs = 0.90, p < 0.01$

*From Sainsbury P, Barraclough, BM: Differences between suicide rates. *Nature* 220:1252, 1968.

confirmed when 24 immigrant groups to Australia were similarly investigated (5, 6). The differences in the incidence of suicide revealed by national mortality statistics were therefore again shown to be valid.

Second, it is objected that statistics are unreliable and suicide is underreported because the criteria of suicide vary from place to place. In particular, many violent deaths, such as those from drowning and poisoning, are more often classified as accidental and of "undetermined cause" in some countries or by some coroners. However, if countries are first ranked in order of their suicide rates and then ranked in order of a rate obtained by combining their suicide, undetermined, and accidental poisoning rates, the two rankings are very significantly alike (Table 2.2) (7, 8). These findings again indicate that the differences between the suicide rates of national and other social groups obtained from official statistics are real and not simply due to methods of ascertainment.

The further allegation that variations in the willingness of coroners (or other officers responsible for recording causes of death) to bring in a verdict of suicide render their figures worthless has also been investigated by correlating the mean suicide rates of the 79 coroners' districts of England and Wales in 1950–1952 and 1960–1962. This procedure was then repeated in those districts in which the coroner had changed during the 10 years and those in which he had not. Table 2.3 shows that the three correlations do not differ appreciably (a district is omitted if a coroner changed during the years from which its mean rate was obtained). It would therefore appear that the idiosyncracies of the coroner are not a source of inaccuracies such as might account for the different incidence of suicide in their districts (4).

Another way of assessing the validity, and hence the value, of mortality rates is to determine whether findings derived from them can be confirmed by other methods, such as by comparing cases of suicide and controls. In an ecological study of suicide in the London boroughs, for example, the suicide rates were found to correlate highly with various indices of social disorganization, isolation, and economic status (such as

Table 2.2. Comparison of the Rank Orders of Mean Suicide Rates per 100,000, and the Combined Suicide, Undetermined, and Accidental Poisoning Death Rates in 19 Countries, 1970 to 1973*, †

Country	Suicide and Self-Inflicted Injury	Rank	Suicide and Self-Inflicted Injury and Injury Undetermined Whether Purposely or Accidentally Inflicted and Accidental Poisoning	Rank
Austria	30.4	4	33.0	6
Bulgaria	15.1	11	19.0	11
Czechoslovakia	31.0	2	39.8	3
Denmark	30.6	3	36.4	4
Finland	29.7	5	40.8	2
France	20.4	9	25.1	9
Germany	26.8	6	29.6	7
Greece	4.1	19	7.1	18
Hungary	45.2	1	48.5	1
Italy	7.6	16	9.2	17
Netherlands	11.3	13	12.9	15
Norway	11.4	12	14.2	14
Poland	15.5	10	23.1	10
Spain	5.9	17	6.8	19
Switzerland	24.6	8	27.2	8
England and Wales	10.3	15	15.5	13
Northern Ireland	5.4	18	11.0	16
Scotland	10.6	14	17.6	12
Sweden	26.4	7	36.0	5

* Data derived from Barraclough (7) and Sainsbury et al (8).
† Spearman's rank correlation = 0.9596, $n = 19$, $p < 0.001$.

Table 2.3. England and Wales: Correlations between (A) Suicide Rates of County Boroughs 1950 to 1952 and 1960 to 1962 with the Same or with a Different Coroner; and (B) Open Verdicts Rates of County Boroughs 1954 to 1957 and 1964 to 1967 with the Same or with a Different Coroner*

Boroughs	No.	Spearman's r	p
A. Suicide rates:			
All	79	0.42	0.001
With same coroner	39	0.45	0.01
With different coroner†	19	0.49	0.05
B. Open verdicts rates:			
Sample	55	0.34	0.02
With same coroner	30	0.56	0.001
With different coroner	20	0.27	N.S.

* Data derived from Sainsbury and Barraclough (4).
† Boroughs in which the coroner changed in the years during which average was estimated are excluded.

the proportion of borough residents who were divorced, illegitimate births, or born outside London). When these statistical associations were tested by using coroners' records to examine the characteristics of the suicides and comparing them with the borough populations at risk, it was possible to confirm many of them (9). Other instances in which case studies have supported a causal hypothesis first suggested by analysis of official statistics will be discussed presently.

The evidence of these very different methods of study is that the mortality statistics are sufficiently accurate to warrant epidemiologists' using the data to see with which national, demographic, social, or other characteristics and their trends they correlate; and thereby not only to test hypotheses about factors predisposing to suicide, but also to identify those groups in a population who are most at risk, and what implications they have for preventive action.

Suicide is underreported for a number of reasons, and the rates are subject to many errors of a kind encountered in reporting mortality figures in general (10). Nevertheless, the findings from studies designed to settle the point indicate that these errors are randomized, at least to an extent that allows epidemiologists profitably to compare rates between countries, within them, and over time.

For all practical epidemiological purposes, underreporting the rate of suicide is of small consequence; while seeking an elusive "absolute" rate by including supposed suicides, such as accidental poisoning deaths (11), only introduces other more serious errors. What matters and what epidemiology seeks to establish is whether differences observed between particular social, clinical, or other categories are valid, because we identify causes and those most at risk by showing that certain groups of people differ consistently in their incidence of suicide.

EXTENT OF THE PROBLEM

Suicide is a major cause of death; it accounts for nearly 1% of all deaths in England and Wales; and though numerically more elderly than young people die by suicide, in 1970 it was the fourth most common cause of death in the age group 15 to 34. It would be reasonable to expect preventive policies to attract the same sort of concern as do automobile accident deaths, which have a comparable mortality.

The overall suicide rate in England in 1980 was 9/100,000 population; the male rate was 12 and the female 8. However, countries differ widely, but consistently, in their incidence of suicide (see Tables 2.1 and 2.2); their rates vary from 2 or 3/100,000 in Ireland to 35 or more in Hungary. In general, the suicide rate is low in the less prosperous Catholic countries and high in the more affluent ones, such as Germany, Switzerland, and Sweden; but it is also high in all Eastern European nations; while the US and Canada, like England, have a rate in the middle range (around 8 to 11/100,000).

Mortality rates for suicide are as a rule higher in urban than in rural districts; indeed suicide has been shown to increase with the size of cities in America (12). Although suicide has a low incidence in closely knit rural communities, the problem increases, especially among the elderly, in areas where agriculture is in decline and workers are emigrating to the cities, as has been happening in the US, Hungary, and Holland (13, 14).

The problem also differs between ethnic and minority groups. The latter often have a lower incidence as is evident when the rates of the black and white populations in the US are compared (14). Minorities tend to bond together in unified communities; and evidence for supposing that social integration protects against suicide will be presented later. Immigrants, on the other hand, have considerably higher rates than both their lost country and their country of origin (see Table 2.1), and those from very different cultures, such as the Chinese and Japanese immigrants to the US, have notably higher rates (14). They are people who are most likely to feel alienated. Suicide varies with the seasons, too, and then more conspicuously in the country than in the city. An increased incidence has been consistently shown in spring and early summer (15), at least in temperate lattitudes. A review of the relations between suicide and the phases of the moon and a wide range of meteorological features conclude that it only varied with the seasons (16). This statistical phenomenon has never been satisfactorily explained; though Durkheim argued that social life intensifies in spring and consequently the alienated become even more bereft.

SEX AND AGE

Figure 2.1 depicts the suicide trends of men and women in England and Wales by 10-year age groups. This pattern is typical of most countries insofar as male rates are consistently higher than female, though in England the difference is less than elsewhere

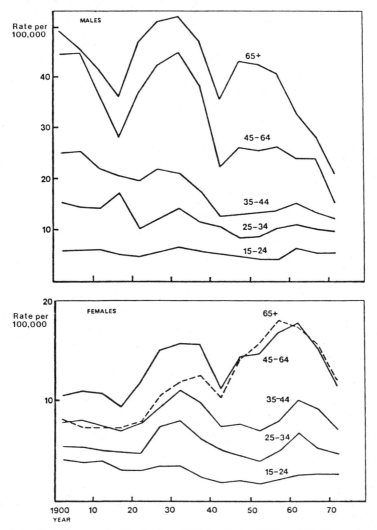

Figure 2.1. Suicide rates in England and Wales from 1900 to 1974 by age and sex. (Adapted from Registrar General: *Statistical Review of England and Wales.*)

Table 2.4. Changes in the Crude Suicide Rate per 100,000 in 18 Countries by Sex, Mean 1961 to 1963 and Mean 1972 to 1974*

	Males			Females			Total (Male & Female)		
	Mean 1961–1963	Mean 1972–1974	% Change	Mean 1961–1963	Mean 1972–1974	% Change	Mean 1961–1963	Mean 1972–1974	% Change
Austria	31.77	32.97	+3.78	13.42	14.23	+6.04	21.88	23.04	+5.30
Belgium	20.39	21.16	+3.78	8.06	9.86	+22.33	14.10	15.39	+9.15
Czechoslo-vakia	29.78	34.98	+17.46	12.36	12.55	+1.54	20.86	23.48	+12.36
Denmark	24.33	31.03	+27.54	12.43	18.24	+46.74	18.33	24.59	+34.15
Finland	33.30	39.08	+17.36	8.96	10.28	+14.73	20.70	23.48	+13.43
France	23.82	22.85	−4.07	7.63	8.93	+17.04	15.50	15.74	+1.55
Germany	25.46	27.19	+6.79	12.94	14.51	+12.13	18.85	20.57	+9.12
Greece	5.05	4.17	−17.43	2.69	1.94	−27.88	3.84	3.03	−21.09
Hungary	36.45	55.14	+51.28	15.65	22.17	+41.66	25.69	38.16	+48.54
Ireland	3.84	5.07	+32.03	1.11	1.75	+57.66	2.48	3.42	+37.90
Italy	7.70	7.88	+2.34	3.27	3.50	+7.03	5.44	5.64	+3.68
Netherlands	8.13	10.29	+26.57	4.86	7.11	+46.30	6.49	8.69	+33.89
Norway	11.66	14.13	+21.18	3.40	4.63	+36.17	7.51	9.35	+24.50
Poland	14.73	19.50	+32.38	3.29	4.23	+28.57	8.83	11.66	+32.05
Sweden	26.78	29.18	+8.96	9.18	11.62	+26.58	17.96	20.36	+13.36
Switzerland	26.42	28.23	+6.85	10.22	11.43	+11.84	18.09	19.64	+8.57
UK England and Wales	14.15	9.38	−33.71	9.58	6.29	−34.34	11.79	7.79	−33.92
Scotland	11.09	9.99	−9.92	6.13	6.68	+8.97	8.51	8.27	−2.82

	Increases = 14			Increases = 16			Increases = 15		
	Decreases = 4			Decreases = 2			Decreases = 3		
	$p = 0.03$			$p = 0.002$			$p = 0.008$		

(Sign test, two-tailed)

* Derived from data in World Health Organization Report (46).

(17–20; Dr Harsluwka, WHO, personal communication, 1975). The trend during this century has been for women's rates to increase nearly everywhere relative to men's. Whereas during the first five decades suicide in men decreased in 8 of 12 European countries, that of women increased in 10 and did not change in 2.

About 1963 suicide in England began to plummet, and this prompted a detailed analysis of the trends in 17 other European countries for the period 1961 to 1974. The suicide rates of *both* sexes had increased in all of them except Greece (and of males in Scotland and France; see Table 2.4), while the ratio of female to male suicide increased still further in most of the 18 countries ($p < 0.01$); the three exceptions were all in Eastern Europe (Hungary, Czechoslovakia, and Poland). The relation between the increasing female rates of suicide and the changing status of women in European societies is discussed below.

Rates of suicide increase with age, though the peak in women is often 10 years earlier than in men (see Fig. 2.2). In England and Scotland during 1961 to 1963 women between 45 and 64 had the highest rate, whereas with men the peaks are at 55 and over. It may be conjectured that the peaks occur at an age when men and women relinquish the principal domestic or occupational roles that society confers on each and they reappraise their purposes in life.

The most distinctive trends of the age- and sex-specific rates in Europe between

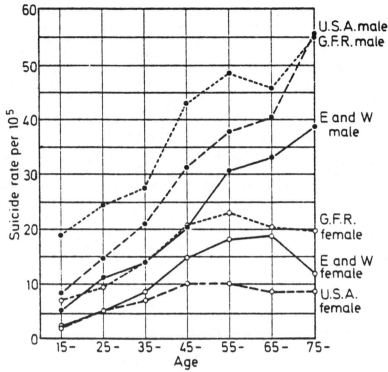

Figure 2.2. Suicide rate per 100,000 by age and sex in the German Federal Republic, England and Wales, and the United States in 1965. (From Sainsbury P: Suicide and attempted suicide. In Kisker K, Meyer J-E, Muller C, Stromgren E (eds): *Psychiatrie der Gegenwart.* Berlin, Springer-Verlag, 1975, pp 557–606.)

1920 and 1954 were (*a*) a *declining* rate in the youths (20 to 39) of both sexes in most of 15 countries; (*b*) increases of suicide in elderly women nearly everywhere, which largely accounts for the rising incidence in women; and (*c*) a decreasing rate in young men in 13 countries (p < 0.02), and in middle age in 10, contributed most to the declining rate of males.

Suicide trends in Europe underwent striking changes during 1961 to 1974 (Dr Harsluwka, WHO, personal communication, 1975). The very sharp decline in England (and to a less extent in Scotland) was apparent in all 10-year age groups for *both* sexes (except women aged 15 to 24), thereby reversing the rising incidence of female suicide which had been evident since 1900; but in the other 17 European countries the opposite occurred. Suicide in women during this period continued to increase, but principally in each 10-year age group between 45 and 74 in a significant proportion of the 18 countries. Though the rate also rose in young women, the increase in young suicides was most marked in men in the age groups 15 to 44 (in men aged 25 to 44 the rise occurred in 15 of the 18 countries). These recent trends in male suicide, particularly in youths, therefore show an impressive departure from those found in the earlier part of this century and provide an objective and poignant indication of the predicament of young people today.

The vulnerability of the aged is also increasing in most of Europe, but especially in women. Epidemiological studies provide hints as to why this should be. Although an increase in suicide with age is general in western societies, exceptions are found in other cultures in which the elders command respect and authority. Figures are scarce, but Modan et al (21) have reported from Israel that whereas Jews of western origin show the usual increase in suicide with aging, those of eastern ethnicity do not. Similarly a rising incidence was not found in Nigeria (22), nor was it apparent in prerevolutionary China (23) when ancestor reverence prevailed and the elderly were held in esteem.

MARITAL STATUS AND FAMILY

Allowing for age, the married have the lowest rates of suicide, then in increasing order are the single, the widowed, the divorced, and the separated; but widowers aged 20 to 25 have an exceptionally high rate (14). Ecological studies also report significant correlations between the suicide and divorce rates of countries and of the districts within them.

More precise case studies comparing suicides from a population and controls matched for age and sex confirm the relationships between marital status and risk and also show that the divorced, and especially the separated, have by far the highest rates. The suicides also had fewer visits from relatives, and the male suicides had fewer children than did the population sample (24). Halbwachs (25) contributed an interesting postscript; he reported that the suicide rate of parents progressively falls as each child is added to the family—but only up to six! Indeed, the rule appears to be that suicide decreases with the number and closeness of the ties within the domestic group and increases with their dissolution, or stated more generally, with the social isolation of members of the family. This view is strongly supported by epidemiological studies that have examined suicides' ties, not only with their family group, but also with their occupational, neighborhood, and religious communities.

SOCIAL RELATIONS OF SUICIDE

Investigations have been of two kinds. First are those in which national mortality figures are related to social statistics derived from the census in order to test a causal association postulated between suicide and selected social variables. Though these studies are economical or relatively simple to do, it is difficult to evaluate the causal direction of the correlations which emerge.

However, positive findings will often justify a second and more arduous method of study, in which consecutive suicides occurring within a census district are identified and their social and other characteristics recorded and compared with those of controls from the general population. This approach combines the advantages of an epidemiological study and a case study.

Neighborhood Ties. The first type of study can be illustrated by the survey of suicides in London (9). The suicide rates of the 28 London boroughs were related to 17 indices of social characteristics of the boroughs which had been postulated as predisposing to suicide. Accordingly, their social isolation was assessed by the proportion of their residents who were living alone and who were immigrants. Both social variables were significantly associated with the boroughs' suicide rates. Next, when coroners' records of some 400 suicides from the boroughs were examined to see whether these relations were probably causal rather than incidental effects, they showed that the suicides indeed lived alone and had been immigrants to a greater extent than the populations at risk.

The pertinence of these social accompaniments of suicide was confirmed in another case study. Barraclough et al (26) interviewed the relatives, friends, and doctors of 100 consecutive suicides dying in West Sussex and Portsmouth and systematically recorded uniform details of their social and medical backgrounds. Similar information was obtained from a sample of the normal population matched on age and sex. The significant differences between the social circumstances of the suicides and controls were much as the social isolation hypothesis predicted. The suicides had fewer ties with their domestic and neighborhood groups when compared with the controls; they found, for example, that more suicides lived alone and also more of them resided in lodgings and hotels, and their relatives lived farther away from them. In addition they had moved house more recently. More of the elderly suicides had retired to the resort towns in the area and had thereby deprived themselves of the support of their previous neighborhood. The suicides' links with family and the local community were therefore fewer than the controls in many respects (6).

Other surveys have compared the suicide rates of districts with differing social characteristics; and, in general, they agree about those that affect incidence. Ashford and Lawrence (27) related the suicide rates of the 170 county boroughs in England and Wales to 88 demographic and social variables recorded in the national census. They found that nearly all of the variance could be explained by very few of their descriptive variables—by far the most important being the proportion of persons living alone. Sakinofsky et al (28) similarly looked at the variation in suicide of the Canadian provinces and found there is a gradient rising from east to west; further analysis using a linear regression of the social variables grouped to provide indices of social and family cohesion showed that most of the variation in male rates of suicide was again accounted for by social isolation and by family disintegration. Ecological studies within cities, notably that of Cavan (29) in Chicago, also showed that the socially mobile and disorganized central districts had the highest incidence of suicide; but unlike the later London studies (9, 30), these areas were also the most destitute, so the separate effects of poverty and of alienation were less readily distinguishable. Lönnqvist (31) in two recent surveys of suicide in Helsinki obtained further support for the hypothesis that suicide relates to measures of social disorganization; he also found that in those areas where social integration had increased between 1961 and 1972, suicide had decreased. Ovenstone (32) observed that the wards in Edinburgh with high rates for child neglect, divorce, and delinquency had the most suicides.

In summary, therefore, alienation and loss of social regulation (anomie) emerge as conditions that predispose to suicide in a variety of social environments.

Religious Affiliations. The suicides documented in Sussex were less involved with the church as well as with their neighborhoods: their attendances were fewer than were those of controls. The protection from suicide afforded by the church is also apparent, or at least suggested, by the low rates reported by those Catholic countries in which religious affiliations are a major influence.

This may be illustrated by an epidemiological digression to consider suicide in Northern Ireland and Eire. In both countries the church is a powerful influence, though Ulster is Protestant and Eire Catholic. Suicide, however, is more specifically proscribed by the latter. Before partition in 1922 their suicide rates were the lowest in Europe; but the rate in Eire was half that of Ulster, and this difference continued after 1922, although both of them still followed the same procedures for ascertaining suicide. It would therefore seem that active religious affiliations may be one factor governing incidence. But what has been less closely examined is the extent to which the church's attitudes toward death, the afterlife, and suicide may account for denominational differences.

Indeed, we know very little about the effect of the differing attitudes of the varied social groups that compose a community on suicide rates. For instance, are the differences in suicide so regularly found between men and women in some measure dependent on their differing notions about death and self-destruction?

CLASS AND OCCUPATIONAL GROUP

The social classes differ in their incidence of suicide; as a rule the higher the social class, whether assessed by income, occupation, or educational attainment, the greater the risk; but a fall in social status also increases it. The relations between poverty, unemployment, and suicide, however, are more complicated.

In England, for example, everyone is allocated at the decennial census to one of five social classes. Table 2.5 depicts a proportional measure (standardized mortality ratio, SMR) of suicide mortality in males (20 to 65) by class at three different periods: relative prosperity, 1921 to 1923; the economic depression, 1930 to 1932; and the postwar period of high employment, 1949 to 1953. It shows that (*a*) the highest SMRs were in the two upper classes and they increased during the economic depression; (*b*) the SMRs in classes 4 and 5 were usually less than 10 and this low level continued in 1930 to 1932, although these classes endured poverty and unemployment at that time; and (*c*) after the war, class 5 became more vulnerable to suicide; unskilled workers had become fewer and this class's composition was determined less by circumstances of birth than previously.

Suicide had a small positive correlation with the social class structure of the London boroughs. This association gains some causal implications when the economic status of the cases of suicide is compared with that of the population at risk: suicide was significantly higher in the middle-class households and lower in those rated as being near the poverty line; but in households below this level the incidence of suicide was twice the expected figure. In Helsinki (31), on the other hand, poverty emerged as a prominent feature of the city districts with a high rate of suicide.

A recent case study comparing the economic status of suicides and matched controls (33) also showed that the two extremes of the social scale had higher rates of suicide. In addition, the authors reported that suicides who were employed were twice as likely as the controls to be in occupations known to have high SMRs for suicide ($p < 0.01$). High risk occupations in England included doctors, lawyers, people in hoteling, nurses, and writers (34).

Table 2.5. England and Wales: Effect of Economic Depression and the Incidence of Suicide in Social Classes (All Males, Aged 20 to 64)*

Social Class	Standardized Mortality Ratio		
	1921–1923 Prosperity	1930–1932 Economic Depression	1949–1953 Welfare State
1. Professional	113	120	140
2. Intermediate between 1 and 3	125	137	113
3. Skilled workers	89	95	89
4. Intermediate between 3 and 5	87	87	92
5. Unskilled workers	96	87	117

* From Registrar General: *Statistical Review of England and Wales*, 1938, 1958.

UNEMPLOYMENT

Ecological studies in Pennsylvania (35), Edinburgh (36), London (9), and 18 European countries (vide infra) all found a very low or negative relationship between districts' rates of suicide and unemployment. But when the more sensitive method of comparing cases and controls from the population is used, it becomes clear that work protects against suicide and lack of work promotes it, a conclusion which Platts (37) also came to in a comprehensive review of unemployment and suicidal behavior. He inferred not only that more suicides are unemployed than would be expected, but also that the unemployed have a higher suicide rate than do the employed. This was clearly borne out in London between 1936 and 1938, where the incidence of unemployment in insured males dying by suicide was 3 times that in the population, and the suicide rate of the unemployed was 5 times the rate in the male population at risk.

When Shepherd and Barraclough (33) compared the work histories of the suicides and matched controls from the same populations, they found that significantly more of the suicides were unemployed. The suicides had also changed jobs more often, held them for a shorter time, and more of them were off work because of illness. Ovenstone (38) commented upon the high incidence of psychiatric disorders among the unemployed in Edinburgh; but when Roy (39) controlled for psychiatric illness, he found that 67% of psychiatrically disturbed suicides were unemployed, whereas only 49% of the psychiatrically ill control patients were.

Whether a predisposition to suicide among the unemployed can be attributed to the effects of lack of work, such as loss of status, of role, and of ties with the working community, or to the concomitant poverty, or to a mental illness precipitated by these stresses (particularly depressive illness)—or, conversely, whether loss of jobs is secondary to personality disorders and illness—remains to be clarified. Meanwhile the probability is that it is a nexus of such considerations which is responsible: an interaction of socioeconomic circumstances, psychological vulnerability, and stressful events.

It would seem that poverty becomes an important factor in suicide according to its context. The indigenous poor, for whom poverty is an accepted feature of their society, tolerate it together. These circumstances do not foster suicide. But a change from comparative affluence to poverty or loss of employment is more disruptive, since the persons affected become alienated and fail to adjust to their altered conditions.

SOCIAL TRENDS AND SUICIDE

Epidemiological inquiries which related changes in suicide rates to social changes (8, 40) and to socioeconomic events can also offer clues to factors affecting the incidence of suicide.

One such study was commissioned by the World Health Organization (WHO) when their mortality statistics showed a surprising decrease in the suicide rate of England and Wales in the early 1960s; evidence of causes responsible for the decline might, it was maintained, provide guides to preventive measures. The investigation showed that suicide in England had fallen by 34% between 1963 and 1974, whereas in all but two European countries suicide had increased during that period. The 18 nations' suicide trends by age and sex were briefly discussed above, and the demographic categories in which the risk had changed most were identified.

When the effects or trends of major socioeconomic events since 1900 are examined, they are seen to be distinctive and consistent (17, 20). In nearly every nation suicide rates rose sharply during the economic depression in the 1930s; whereas they fell during both world wars, the effects being more marked on men than women, and the English figures show that middle-aged men were especially affected (Tables 2.6 and 2.7, Fig. 2.1).

These observations clearly indicate that social events do, in fact, affect national rates of suicide, sometimes by as much as 50%, and that demographic groups are differentially influenced. In particular, the consistency with which trends of suicide in women, the young, and the aged are changing and are modified by social and political vicissitudes argues strongly that there is scope for preventive action at the social level.

The authors therefore examined a number of hypothetical explanations for the exceptional decline in England. That it could be attributed to statistical inaccuracies arising from the procedures for ascertaining suicide was ruled out, nor did changes in the criteria for defining suicide have any effect. For example, suicide ceased to be a criminal offense in 1961, and the *International Classification of Diseases* introduced a new category—"undetermined" whether cause of death was suicide or accident—in 1967. In the former instance the mean suicide rate for 3 years after 1961 increased

Table 2.6. Changes in the Incidence of Suicide by Sex and Age in Selected Countries between 1921 to 1922 and 1931 to 1932 (Economic Depression) (Percentage Change—Mortality around 1920 to 1921 = 100)*

Country	Males			Females		
	20–39	40–49	60+	20–39	40–49	60+
South Africa	+10	−4	+17	+63	+104	+35
Canada	+29	+48	+33	+32	+15	+23
Chile	+96	+150	+41	+90	+200	N.K.
United States	+6	+28	+36	+19	+21	+20
Germany	−3	+17	+1	+13	+28	+15
Belgium	+29	+19	+19	−6	+18	+2
Denmark	+13	+22	−9	+88	+6	+5
Spain	−5	+36	+23	+14	+26	+33
Finland	+108	+58	+68	+39	+42	+13
France	+8	+3	0	−5	+5	−5
Italy	+5	+76	+55	−4	+47	+52
Norway	+22	+35	+49	+63	+18	−24
Netherlands	−14	+11	−1	+15	+54	+38
Portugal	+14	+61	+54	−10	+5	+46
England and Wales	+41	+20	+16	+42	+32	+45
Scotland	+56	+77	+76	+128	+91	+68
Sweden	−9	+8	−2	+3	−2	−15
Switzerland	+13	+5	+5	−4	+13	−9
Australia	+25	+10	0	0	+17	−7
New Zealand	−10	+26	+19	−5	+28	+47
No. which increased	15	19	15	13	19	14
No. which decreased	5	1	3	6	1	5
No change or no. not known	0	0	2	1	0	1
Sign test, two-tailed *p*	0.042	<0.001	0.008	0.168	<0.001	0.064
No. of times age group had:						
Greatest increase	6	11	3	5	10	5
Greatest decrease	5	1	1	4	0	4

* Adapted from World Health Organization Report (17) and Sainsbury (20).

Table 2.7. Effect of War on Suicide Rates by Sex in Selected Belligerent and Neutral Countries (Suicides per 100,000 Population Aged 15 and Over)*

Country	Male			Female		
	1938	1944	Percentage Difference	1938	1944	Percentage Difference
Belligerent countries						
Union of South Africa	15.5	10.7	−31	5.0	3.4	−32
Canada	13.1	8.9	−32	3.7	3.2	−14
United States	23.5	14.9	−37	6.9	5.4	−22
Ceylon	10.1	8.2	−19	3.9	4.1	+5
Austria†	60.7	28.1	−54	28.6	13.8	−52
France	31.0	18.2	−41	8.9	6.1	−31
Italy	11.0	6.0	−45	3.6	2.0	−44
England and Wales	18.0	13.5	−25	8.2	5.8	−29
Scotland	12.3	9.1	−26	6.3	4.5	−29
North Ireland	6.9	5.6	−19	6.9	5.6	−18
Australia	16.4	9.9	−40	5.0	4.9	−2
New Zealand	19.5	14.6	−25	5.1	5.7	+12
Belgium	27.6	18.1	−34	8.6	6.5	−24
Denmark	28.9	24.0	−17	12.9	20.5	+59
Finland	32.8	27.7	−16	7.3	5.3	−27
Norway	10.7	8.2	−23	5.3	9.8	+85
Netherlands	11.6	7.4	−36	5.4	5.6	+4
Japan‡	21.0	18.7	−11	12.9	12.9	0
Neutral countries						
Chile	6.8	6.5	−4	2.5	2.3	−8
Ireland	4.7	4.6	−2	1.8	0.6	−67
Portugal	16.6	13.9	−16	5.0	4.8	−4
Sweden	25.0	20.6	−18	6.8	5.7	−16
Switzerland	38.4	37.2	−3	11.6	14.7	+27
Spain§	6.9	8.8	+28	2.3	2.6	+13

* Data derived from World Health Organization Report (17) and Sainsbury (20).
† Nearest figures available for Austria were for 1946.
‡ Nearest figures available for Japan were for 1947; Japan was also at war in 1938.
§ Civil war in Spain in 1938.

slightly in women, but decreases in men compared with the previous 3 years; as regards the latter, the trends of the suicide rates by age and sex and those of an "estimated" rate of suicide obtained by adding accidental and undetermined deaths to the suicides were virtually parallel.

Second, changes in the availability of the means of committing suicide were invoked. On the one hand, domestic gas, which was the favored method of suicide in England, was being rendered harmless in 1960, and, on the other, the increasing ease with which hypnotics could be obtained in most countries might have accounted for their rising rates; but the evidence lent little support for these contentions (see "The Epidemiology of Methods of Suicides," below). The third hypothesis, that the reduction in England's suicide rate could be ascribed to improvement in the primary care services, was only borne out in part (see Chapter 5).

A fourth explanation postulated that the decline in suicide in Britain and its increases elsewhere in Europe related to social and economic changes between 1961 and 1974.

Social Relations of Suicide Trends in Europe, 1961 to 1963 and 1972 to 1974

Durkheim (41) maintained that suicide increases as cohesion within the society diminishes or when society's control over its members is reduced ("anomie"). To test these concepts they need to be restated in operational terms by selecting national statistics that describe the social conditions which he postulated as predisposing to suicide.

To do this the mean values of 15 social variables from 18 countries for the years 1961 to 1963 and 1972 to 1974 were obtained (8, 42). Table 2.8 lists the variables and the social factors they are intended to describe: some are presumed to be indicators of anomie and some of socioeconomic status, while others refer to demographic groups in the population which have been identified as having become more vulnerable to suicide, e.g., measures of women's changing status and of the alienation of the young and elderly. In Table 2.9 the 18 countries are ranked in order of the change in their mean suicide rates during the two periods and are then split at the median to provide two groups: countries whose suicide rates decreased or only increased a little, and those in which the increase was substantial.

The mean suicide rates of the 18 countries were then correlated to each of the social variables separately during the initial period (1961 to 1963) to identify possible determinants of suicide; next the *changes* in rates of suicide between 1961 and 1974

Table 2.8. Selected Social Variables and the Social Processes They Describe

Social Variable	Social Indicators of				
	Anomie	Family Cohesion	Status of Women	Alienation of Aged	Socioeconomic Status
1. Percentage of population under 15 years	x	x	x	x	
2. Percentage of population aged 65+		x		x	
3. Marriage rate	x	x	x		
4. Divorce rate	x	x	x		
5. Illegitimacy	x	x	x		
6. Births to women under 20		x	x		
7. Births to women over 30		x	x		
8. Women in tertiary education			x		
9. Female employment			x		
10. TV sets/100,000 population					x
11. Room occupancy					x
12. Unemployment	x				x
13. Cirrhosis of liver deaths	x				
14. Homocide rate	x				
15. Road accident death rate	x				

Table 2.9. Change in Mean Suicide Rates for Overall Population 1961 to 1963 and 1972 to 1974 of 18 Countries Ranked in Order

	Rank		%	
Group 1 (Low)	1.	England and Wales	−33.9	⎫
	2.	Greece	−21.1	⎬ Decline
	3.	Scotland	−2.8	⎭
	4.	France	1.6	
	5.	Italy	3.7	
	6.	Austria	5.3	
	7.	Switzerland	8.6	
	8.	Germany	9.1	
	9.	Belgium	9.2	
Group 2 (High)	10.	Czechoslovakia	12.6	
	11.5	Finland	13.4	
	11.5	Sweden	13.4	
	13.	Norway	24.5	
	14.	Poland	32.1	
	15.	Netherlands	33.9	
	16.	Denmark	34.2	
	17.	Ireland	37.9	
	18.	Hungary	48.5	

were correlated with *changes* in the social variables. Multivariate analyses were undertaken to determine what combination of social variables differentiated the countries with a rising suicide rate from those with a falling rate.

Correlation between 18 Countries' Suicide Rates and 15 Social Variables

Sainsbury et al. (40) found that significant correlations between the suicide rates and social variables were in accordance with previous ecological studies of districts *within* a country or city. Thus, suicide related inversely to measures of family cohesion: the proportion of the population aged less than 15, and births to women over 30. Suicide also related strongly to indicators of "anomie": rates of divorce and illegitimacy. The novel indices of women's status in the countries, their employment rates, and births to women below 20, were significantly associated with suicide; whereas two of the socioeconomic measures varied inversely, but weakly with suicide, which is again in accordance with previous observations. These associations were much the same for men as for women.

When the effects of *changes* in the social variables on suicide were examined the findings were as they had predicted. Suicide again rose concurrently with increases in the measures of anomie; and increasing affluence, as measured by rising rates of television ownership, was also accompanied by more suicide. As regards the changing role of women, an important finding was that suicide in both sexes increased with the number of employed women.

Multivariate Analysis

The problem of obtaining a more coherent view of the interaction between suicide and a social environment which is changing in many respects can be more appropriately unraveled by multivariate analysis.

Discriminant function is one technique by which to assess the relative contributions the set of variables (the social measures) makes to allocating the countries to the previously determined classification, namely, the changes in 18 countries' suicide rates when ranked and split at the median to provide two groups. The 15 social variables were therefore used to predict the likelihood that a given country will fall into group 1 in which suicide had decreased or only shown a small increase, or group 2 in which suicide increased substantially. (The predicted order could then also be compared with observed order). The analysis also classified each social variable according to its discriminating power (the DF coefficient).

Table 2.10, for example, shows the extent to which the initial values of the combined social measures correctly predicted the changes in the countries' suicide rates in the following 10 years. All the countries are correctly classified into group 1 or group 2; but within the groups some countries' predicted rank positions differ from the observed ones. The variables which contributed most to the discrimination were (*a*) those that relate to number of children and pattern of childbirth, and (*b*) socioeconomic ones. Similarly, when the *changes* in the social variables during the 10 years were applied to the changes in the suicide rates, the analysis again correctly classified each country according to whether suicide decreased or increased. Indicators of the changing status of women (rates of marriage, females in education and in employment) contributed most to the discrimination. The other important variable, whose increase determined the extent to which a country's suicide increased, was unemployment.

The value of various social measures, selected because of their supposed pertinence in predisposing to suicide, therefore enabled each country to be correctly grouped according to whether its suicide rate would rise or fall.

Table 2.10. Discriminate Function Analysis: Number 1. Part A: Change in Overall Suicide Rate by Base Rates of the Social Variables in 1961 to 1963*

Countries	Rank Order of Suicide Rates		Discriminant Function Score
	Predicted	Observed	
Group 1 (Low)			
Germany†	1	8	6.04
France	2	4	6.03
Greece	3	2	5.73
Scotland	4	3	5.65
Italy	5	5	5.34
England and Wales‡	6	1	5.24
Switzerland	7	7	5.11
Austria	8	6	4.36
Belgium	9	9	3.26
Group 2 (High)			
Denmark†	10	15	3.28
Norway	11	13	3.75
Ireland†	12	17	4.84
Finland	13	11.5	4.90
Czechoslovakia‡	14	10	5.46
Poland	15	14	5.99
Sweden†	16	11.5	6.00
Netherlands	17	16	6.26
Hungary	18	18	6.27

* Canonical correlation = 0.98 (correlation between suicide and composite variable).
† Actual rank much higher.
‡ Actual rank much lower.

Because discriminant function may be criticized when there are 15 social variables and only 18 countries, the authors also undertook a *multiple regression analysis* using a technique developed by Furnival and Wilson (43) to select the best set of 4 or 5 predictors from the 15 possibilities. The first aim of this analysis was to assess the extent to which the *initial* values of the selected social variables, when combined, would accurately predict the *changes* in the suicide rates of the 18 countries between 1961 and 1974.

They identified the mean values (in 1961 to 1963) of the following five social variables as the best predictors: the countries' rates of divorce, unemployment, homicide, and women in employment, and the percentage of the population over the age of 15. This selected set of predictors was then entered into the regression analysis.

Figure 2.3 shows how closely the predicted changes in the countries' suicide rates resemble their observed changes. What is also of interest is the precision with which the decline in suicide in England and Greece is anticipated and hinted at if not explained (42).

They next obtained an additional set of four variables to describe the *social changes* in each country over the 10 years and entered it into a second regression analysis. Figure 2.4 lists the selected variables and again shows how accurately the changes in their values predicted changes in the 18 countries' rates of suicide (42).

Despite the limited choice of appropriate social statistics for all of Europe and the lack of data on such relevant considerations as indices of social isolation (numbers of immigrants or of persons living alone, for instance), the statistics which are available gave surprisingly exact predictions of the increases and decreases of suicide in Europe. What also clearly emerges is both the extent to which changing social conditions affect national trends in suicide and the consistency with which certain socioeconomic

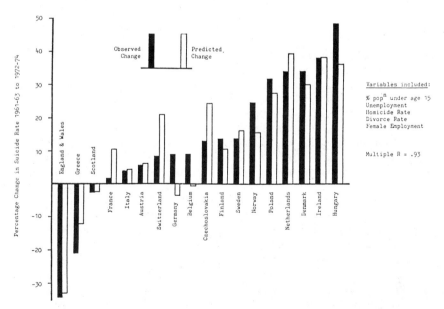

Figure 2.3. Observed and predicted changes in the suicide rates of 18 European countries between 1961 ato 1963 and 1972 to 1974. Results of multiple regression analysis, using base values of social variables.

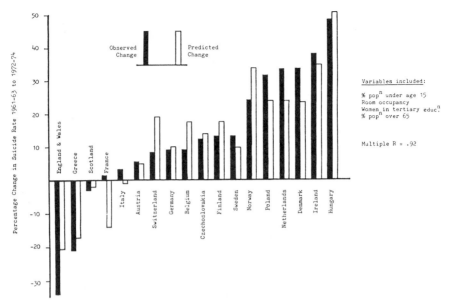

Figure 2.4. Observed and predicted changes in the suicide rates of 18 European countries between 1961 to 1963 and 1972 to 1974. Results of multiple regression analysis, using percentage changes in social variables between 1961 to 1963 and 1972 to 1974.

developments, notably unemployment and women's roles in society, contribute to its incidence.

THE EPIDEMIOLOGY OF METHODS OF SUICIDES

The means used to commit suicide can be most profitably considered in the context of suicide prevention, or more precisely by asking whether ease of access to a given method can affect the *incidence* of suicide rather than simply the *proportion* of suicides who use one method in preference to another. For example, in England and Wales about 1960, carbon monoxide poisoning was the favored method; it accounted for nearly 50% of all suicides. At this time detoxified or natural gas was introduced, and a steep decline in the suicide rate coincided with the decrease in the carbon monoxide content of domestic gas. First Hassell and Trethowan (44) and then Kreitman (45) argued that the nonlethal gas accounted for the sudden fall in the number of suicides.

Before investigating this claim, the WHO statistics on the methods used by suicides in 12 countries during 1955 to 1969 warrant examination (46). These make it clear that to some extent availability determines the means chosen. For example, firearms are the commonly used methods in gun-carrying nations such as the US, and incidentally among rural populations; carbon monoxide is most often used in coal-producing nations; drowning is more frequently favored in the watery Netherlands. In general, however, hanging is the most widely used of all. But preferences change with circumstances; carbon monoxide poisoning has fallen sharply nearly everywhere (though the use of automobile exhaust gas is increasing); while poisoning with medicinals has increased in 11 of the 12 European countries; poisoning is now the principal method in 3 of them.

Social custom also affects choice. Suicides in most countries continue to prefer a particular means, and evidence for this is apparent when the methods used by immigrants are compared with those of their host country (47).

Last, when methods are examined by age and sex, men everywhere favor the more violent methods and women more passive ones. By 1969, for instance, poisoning had become the means most often used by women in 8 of 12 countries; the young are now also turning to medicinals, but the elderly still adhere to the traditional hanging.

The widespread and increasing use of drugs again raises the question of whether their easy availability can, in part, explain the recent increase in the suicide rates of so many nations.

Domestic Gas and Suicide. Barraclough tested the view that suicide in England has declined with the diminishing lethality of domestic gas by comparing the suicide rates in 1958 and 1967 of a group of towns where the carbon monoxide content of gas was reduced below the lethal level in 1967 with a group of towns where it remained lethal in both periods. The two groups were closely matched on their suicide rates in 1958–before detoxification—but in 1967 the suicide rates of both sets of towns had decreased by the same amount (see Table 2.11).

A second and similarly designed study compared two larger groups of county boroughs, but over a shorter period. Suicide decreased by 18% in the 9 boroughs in which the carbon monoxide level had been reduced to a low level between 1968 and 1966, and by 14% in the 15 boroughs where the level remained lethal; this difference was not significant (8).

These controlled comparisons suggest that the association between the fall in suicide and carbon monoxide content of domestic gas may have been coincidental rather than causal, and that other factors are lowering the suicide rate in Britain.

Further evidence was sought in Holland, because carbon monoxide poisoning was the second most frequent method of suicide there and the Dutch were also replacing coal gas with harmless natural gas, particularly because, in contrast to that in England,

Table 2.11. Changes in Suicide Rates per Million Population in Two Groups of County Boroughs: One with a High and the Other with a Low Content in Carbon Monoxide in Domestic Gas in 1967, but below 5% after 1967

County Boroughs	1958			1967			Change in Rate*
	Suicides	Population	Suicide Rate	Suicides	Population	Suicide Rate	
Group A: Mean CO in 1967 = 16.2%							
Southampton	20	199,000	101	29	210,000	138	+37
Ipswich	9	113,000	80	11	122,000	90	+10
Coventry	32	281,000	114	34	334,000	102	−12
Carlisle	8	69,000	116	6	71,000	85	−31
Gloucester	9	68,000	132	9	85,000	106	−26
Exeter	12	77,000	156	8	93,000	86	−70
Total	90	807,000	112	97	915,000	106	−6
Group B: Mean CO in 1967 <5%							
Darlington	9	83,000	108	14	85,000	165	+57
Tynemouth	5	69,000	72	8	72,000	111	+39
Norwich	18	119,000	151	14	119,000	118	−33
South Shields	13	109,000	119	9	108,000	83	−36
Total	45	380,000	118	45	384,000	117	−1

* Mann-Whitney test: $U = 21$, $p = <0.05$.

the Dutch suicide rate was rising. Moreover, when this rising trend was examined by methods of suicide, the fall in the carbon monoxide suicide rate was wholly compensated by an increase in the drug suicide rate, an observation which is contrary to what might be expected by those who attribute the falling suicide in England to the lack of lethal domestic gas.

With the help of the Dutch Central Bureau of Statistics (Dutch Inspectorate of Mental Health, personal communication, 1977), the Medical Research Council's team looked at the changes in the suicide rates of six Dutch provinces in which the sales of gas containing carbon monoxide had fallen to a relatively harmless level between 1960 and 1965 and compared them with the changes in the rates of the three provinces where the domestic gas sold was still lethal in 1965. They found that the suicide rate rose by 14% in the former province and by 4% in the latter. This difference is significant ($p < 0.025$), but in the opposite direction to that which would be expected by those who postulate that rendering domestic gas harmless can lower the suicide rate to the extent recorded in England.

Nevertheless, the same may not be true as regards the effect of hypnotic and other potentially lethal drugs on suicide. The majority of suicides dying from an overdose had taken barbiturates (48). Between 1962 and 1972, however, the rate of prescribing barbiturates/100 population fell by about 37% (49). This might have been expected to have led to fewer deaths, but the *proportion* of suicides taking barbiturates and the barbiturate suicide rate rose during that decade. On the other hand, in Sweden where suicide is increasing, both the prescribing of barbiturates and the number of suicides taking them have fallen, so in neither country had the reduction in availability of this drug had an appreciable impact on incidence.

The decline in suicide in England could also have arisen because more deaths are from poisoning so that the cautious coroner now has more opportunity to allocate poisoning deaths to accidental or undetermined causes rather than to suicide. However, the ratio of suicides by poisoning to undetermined and accidental deaths by poisoning actually increased between 1961 and 1972 instead of falling (50).

A critical examination of mortality statistics therefore supports the notion that when intending suicides are deprived of access to a means of committing the act, they return to other methods, so that measures taken to limit availability, such as converting to natural gas or restricting the prescription of drugs, are unlikely to lower incidence or contribute substantially to suicide prevention.

Life Events and Suicide

Barraclough (51) also obtained details of the recent stressful life events encountered by a sample of 75 suicides (by interviewing relatives and friends) and 150 matched controls. The suicides experienced more events than did the controls. The number of stresses they endured were more than would be expected by chance and included money and legal problems, illness in the family, and loss of job. However, the more conspicuous events were bereavement and moving house, and physical illnesses also merit comment.

Bereavement

A recent bereavement was a prominent stress which preceded suicide. Bunch et al (52) found that suicides had suffered the recent loss of a parent to a much greater extent that had the age-matched normal population; moreover, certain psychiatric and family characteristics affected the likelihood of suicide following bereavement. Sixty percent of the bereaved, for example, had a history of previous mental illness; and males who had lost their mothers were more at risk, especially if they were unmarried. On the other hand, and contrary to some opinions, they obtained no evidence that early parental bereavement (before the age of 16) had an effect on the risk of suicide. McMahon and Pugh (53) showed the risk is also increased in the 4 years following the loss of a spouse; in the case of maternal bereavement the risk was greatest in the 3 years after her death ($p < 0.01$).

Moving House

Reference has already been made to the finding that the proportion of residents of the London boroughs who are foreign immigrants and those who are immigrants from other parts of England both correlate highly with the boroughs' suicide rates. When Barraclough and Warnke later related the suicide rates of 83 country boroughs to the duration of residence of men and women, female suicide correlated highly in each of the first 5 years; whereas women who still lived in the towns where they were born had a significantly reduced rate of suicide. The relationship was less pronounced for men, though moving house and suicide correlated significantly at 5 years. However, these statistical associations do not resolve the problem of causation.

They become clearer when suicides and controls who moved home are compared: a much higher percentage of suicides than the normal population had moved in the previous 2 years. Moreover, the suicides who had moved were more isolated than either the controls or the suicides who had not moved house: more of them were single or widowed, living alone, childless, and without relatives nearby than could be accounted for by chance (6).

When the suicides who had moved were divided into those who moved once or not at all and those who had made a number of moves, the latter were differentiated by more of them having an abnormal personality, being alcoholics, making more previous suicide attempts, and having more encounters with the law. In short, they are the suicides who are recruited from those asocial personalities who make repeated attempts and eventually succeed. Nearly all of the other groups of suicides had a depressive illness.

Physical Illness

A widely held opinion is that physical illness and disabilities are misfortunes that commonly precipitate suicide; but this is not borne out when the medical histories, physical conditions, and postmortems of the suicides were independently assessed by a consultant physician and compared with matched controls admitted to hospital for minor surgery. The two groups did not differ with respect to serious and malignant illness, though the suicides had made more complaints of a minor kind in the period preceding their death. The position regarding mental illness and suicide is very different however (see Chapter 9).

CONCLUSION

These examples of the uses of the epidemiology of suicide are far from complete, relying as they do to a considerable extent on the experiences and research of the author and his colleagues. Their purpose, however, is not so much to present a comprehensive review as to illustrate how epidemiological methods can be applied to investigate factors that predispose to suicide. The potential value of such inquiries extends beyond attaining a better understanding of suicide because, as was suggested earlier, suicide is unique among the behavioral abnormalities of man in being the one aberration for which extensive and international statistical data are available and which invite the attention of research sociologists and behavioral scientists.

By exploring the official mortality reports, census and survey findings that most developed countries publish, and then deriving suicide rates for diverse demographic and social categories, those groups of people who are most vulnerable can be identified. It then becomes feasible to propose explanations for the differences found between them and plan studies to test them. Similarly, these data enable us to examine trends and so distinguish those conditions that relate to increases or decreases in mortality, as was attempted, for instance when explanations were sought for the decline in suicide in England.

Besides their contribution to the natural history of suicide, this type of inquiry is of particular value in assessing the effects of preventative measures and therapeutic innovations.

More importantly, if those who are most prone to suicide, and the circumstances and conditions which foster it, can be identified by epidemiological studies, there is the real scope for devising practical preventive policies both at the grass-root and governmental levels; and this surely should be the major goal of suicide research.

References

1. Sainsbury P: The social relations of suicide. *Soc Sci Med* 6:198, 1972.
2. Douglas JD: *The Social Meaning of Suicide.* Princeton, Princeton University Press, 1967.
3. Atkinson MW, Kessel, Dalgaard JB: The comparability of suicide rates. *Br J Psychiatry* 127:247, 1975.
4. Sainsbury P, Barraclough BM: Differences between suicide rates. *Nature* 220:1252, 1968.
5. Lester D: Letter. *Med J Aust* 941, 1972.
6. Sainsbury P: Suicide: opinions and facts. *Proc R Soc Med* 66:579, 1973.
7. Barraclough BM: Differences between national suicide rates. *Bri J Psychiatry* 122:95, 1973.
8. Sainsbury P, Jenkins JS, Levey A, Baert A: Suicide trends in Europe: a study of the decline in suicide in England and Wales and the increase elsewhere. Geneva, WHO Regional Office for Europe, 1978.
9. Sainsbury P: *Suicide in London.* Maudsley Monograph no. 1. London, Chapman and Hall, 1955.
10. General Register Office: Studies on medical and population subject, no. 20. Accuracy of certification of cause of death. London, Her Majesty's Stationery Office, 1966.
11. Adelstein A, Mardon C: Suicides 1961–1974. Population trends, no. 2, London, OPCS, Her Majesty's Stationery Office, 1975, p 13.
12. Dublin LI, Bunzel BC: *To Be or Not To Be, a Study of Suicide.* New York, Random House, 1933.
13. Gargas S: Suicide in Netherlands. *Am J Sociol* 37:697, 1932.
14. Kramer M, Pollack ES: *Mental Disorders: Suicide.* Cambridge, MA, Harvard University Press, 1972.
15. Barraclough BM, White S: Monthly variation of suicide and undetermined death compared. *Br J Psychiatry* 132:275, 1978.
16. Pokorny A: Myths about suicide. In Resnick H (ed): *Suicidal Behaviors, Diagnosis and Management.* Boston, Little, Brown, and Co, 1968.
17. World Health Organization: *Epidemiology and Vital Statistics,* Report 9, no. 4. Geneva, World Health Organization, 1956.
18. World Health Organization: *Epidemiology and Vital Statistics,* Report 14, no 5. Geneva, World Health Organization, 1961.
19. World Health Organization: *World Health Statistics,* Report 21, no. 6. Geneva, World Health Organization, 1968.

20. Sainsbury P: Social and epidemiological aspects of suicide with special references to the aged. In Williams RH, Tibbitts C, Donahue W (eds): *Processes of Ageing.* Atherton Press, New York, 1963, vol 2.
21. Modan B, Nissenkorn I, Lewkowski SR: Suicide in a heterogenous society. *Br J Psychiatry* 126:301, 1970.
22. Asuni T: Suicide in Western Nigeria. *Br Med J* 2: 1091, 1962.
23. Yap PM: Ageing and mental illness in Hong Kong. In Williams RH, Tibbitts C, Donahue W (eds): *Processes of Ageing.* Atherton Press, New York, 1963, vol 2.
24. Barraclough BM, Nelson B: Marriage and suicide. Society for Psychosomatic Research, 15th Annual Conference, London, 1974.
25. Halbwachs M: *The Causes of Suicide.* Paris, Felix Alcar, 1930.
26. Barraclough BM, Bunch J, Nelson B, Sainsbury P: A hundred cases of suicide: clinical aspects. *Br J Psychiatry* 125:355, 1974.
27. Ashford JR, Lawrence PA: Aspects of the epidemiology of suicide in England and Wales. *Int J Epidemiol* 5:133, 1976.
28. Sakinofsky I, Roberts R, Vartbuten A: Paper presented at the International Congress of Suicide Prevention, Jerusalem, 1975.
29. Cavan RS: *Suicide.* Chicago, University of Chicago Press, 1928.
30. Whitlock FA: Suicide in England and Wales 1959–63. *Psychol Med* 3: 1973.
31. Lönnqvist J: Suicide in Helsinki. *Monogr Psychiatr Fenn,* no. 8, 1977.
32. Ovenstone IMK: A psychiatric approval to the diagnosis of suicide and its effects on the Edinburgh statistics. *Br J Psychiatry* 123:15, 1978.
33. Shepherd DM, Barraclough BM: Work and suicide—an empirical investigation. *Br J Psychiatry* 136:469, 1980.
34. Registrar General: *Occupational Mortality Tables 1961.* London, Her Majesty's Stationery Office, 1971.
35. Walbran B, McMahon B, Bailey AE: Suicide and unemployment in Pennsylvania, 1954–61. *Arch Environ Health* 10:11, 1965.
36. Buglass D, Duffy JC: The ecological pattern of suicide and parasuicide in Edinburgh. *Soc Sci Med* 12:241, 1978.
37. Platts S: Unemployment and suicidal behavior—a review of the literature. *Soc Sci Med* 19:93–115, 1984.
38. Ovenstone IMK: Spectrum of suicidal behavior in Edinburgh. *Br J Prev Soc Med* 126:301, 1973.
39. Roy A: Risk factors for suicide in psychiatric patients. *Arch Gen Psychiatry* 39:1089, 1982.
40. Sainsbury P, Jenkins JP, Levey A: The social correlates of suicide in Europe. In Farmer R, Hirsch S (eds): *The Suicide Syndrome.* London, Croom Helm, 1980.
41. Durkheim E: *Le Suicide: Etude de Sociologie.* Paris, Felix Alcan, 1897.
42. Jenkins JS: Doctoral thesis: An ecological examination of the social relations of the suicide rate changes of 18 European countries 1961–63 to 1972–74. Sussex University, 1984.
43. Furnival GM, Wilson RW: Regression by leaps and bounds. *Technometrics* 16:479, 1974.
44. Hassell C, Trethowan W: Suicide in Birmingham. *Br Med J* 1:717, 1972.
45. Kreitman N: The coal-gas story: UK suicide rates 1960–1971. *Br J Prev Soc Med* 30:86, 1976.
46. World Health Organization: *World Health Statistics Report,* 26, no. 3. Geneva, World Health Organization, 1973.
47. Whitlock FA: Migration and suicide. *Med J Aust* 11: 840, 1971.
48. Barraclough BM: Suicide and barbiturate prescribing. *J R Coll Gen Practitioners* 21:645, 1971.
49. Johns MW: Self poisoning with barbiturates in England and Wales during 1959–1974. *Br Med J* 1:1128, 1977.
50. Sainsbury P, Jenkins JS: The accuracy of officially reported suicide statistics for purposes of epidemiological research. *J Epidemiol Community Health* 56:48, 1982.
51. Barraclough BM: Life events preceding suicide. In Proceedings of Conference on Social Psychiatry, Opatija, 1975.

52. Bunch J, Barraclough BM, Nelson B, Sainsbury P: Suicide following bereavement of parents. *Soc Psychiatry* 6:193, 1971.
53. McMahon B, Pugh TF: Suicide in the widowed. *Am J Epidemiol*, 81:23, 1965.
54. Registrar General: *Statistical Review of England and Wales.* Deceminal Supplement 1931, part IIa. London, Her Majesty's Stationery Office, 1938.
55. Registrar General: *Statistical Review of England and Wales.* London, Her Majesty's Stationery Office, 1958.

3

Genetic Factors in Suicide

Seymour S. Kety, M.D.

Suicide is an example of deviant behavior where both environmental and genetic factors may be important or necessary, and neither alone may be sufficient. The literature over many years has cited a large number of socioenvironmental factors which are associated with suicide (1), and several chapters in this volume deal with these influences in great detail. There are marked differences in the rates for suicide according to age, religion, the country in which the study is carried out, and the particular period in that country's history. For example, in the United States there has been a striking increase in adolescent suicides in the past two decades. Such marked variations cannot be explained on the basis of genetic variance because the genes do not vary so widely from one country to another, nor do they vary within a country from one time to another. There are also personal factors associated with suicide: marital status, financial circumstances, unemployment, parental loss, and others which inlfuence the risk. In addition, there are important psychiatric risk variables, especially a previous history or concurrent presence of depression or schizophrenia (2, 3).

The plausibility that significant cultural influences and devastating personal experiences could cause suicide, at a time when single causes sufficed for explanations, diminished the motivation to seek other types of influence. The "nature versus nurture" question, now thought to be obsolete, appeared to be settled in favor of environmental factors.

Hypotheses suggesting the operation of genetic influences in suicide were infrequently proposed and inadequately examined. Although families with a high incidence of suicide were known and sometimes reported in the literature, this could be explained on the basis of cultural and psychological attributes shared by a family without invoking their genetic endowment. It was to be expected that genetic factors if present in suicide would be clearly demonstrated by studies on twins, and it was therefore very significant that Franz Kallmann, who found high concordance rates for schizophrenia and manic-depressive illness in monozygotic twins, found no concordance at all for suicide (4), concluding that genetic factors did not operate significantly in that behavioral deviance.

Twenty years later, however, Haberlandt (5), reviewing later studies, found an 18% concordance rate for suicide in a total of 51 monozygotic twin pairs and no dizygotic twins concordant for suicide. More recently, Juel-Nielsen and Videbech (6) found a significant number of concordant monozygotic twin pairs with suicide. In no series is the concordance rate as high as it is for depression or schizophrenia; this is probably because the risk of suicide itself in the population is quite low compared to that of schizophrenia or manic-depressive illness. Furthermore, an environmental stressor

41

which may have been a necessary contributing factor to the suicide of one twin may not have been present in the experience of the other. It is also possible that suicide in one twin actually diminishes the possibility of suicide in the remaining twin through psychological mechanisms.

Because of the obvious ways in which suicidal risk and behavior in twins and in members of a family could be enhanced or attenuated by psychological interactions between them, studies in adopted individuals and their biological and adoptive relatives with respect to attempted and completed suicide are of interest. Two such studies have been completed, both utilizing a national sample of individuals legally adopted in Denmark between 1925 and 1948. Because of the excellent adoption and population records maintained in that country (7), as the basis of one study it was possible to identify the biological and adoptive parents, siblings, and half-siblings of a proband group consisting of 57 adoptees who had committed suicide (8). For the second study (9), 71 adoptees who had suffered a depressive illness were selected. For each study, an equal number of matched control adoptees were selected, and searches were made of vital statistics and hospital records for evidence of attempted or completed suicide in their biological or adoptive relatives.

The results of the study by Schulsinger et al (8) are presented in Table 3.1. In the biological relatives of the adoptees who had committed suicide there was a 4.5% incidence of suicide compared to an incidence of less than 1% in the biological relatives of the controls. There were no suicides in the adoptive relatives of either group. The psychiatric register was searched for indications of depression or other mental illness in those relatives who had committed suicide. In approximately 50%, no such history was found. Although that does not exclude the possibility that a brief period of depression could have preceded the suicide, it was suggested that there is a type of suicide which is not necessarily associated with mental illness.

The prevalence of suicide in relatives of adoptees selected for depression, and of their control adoptees from the study of Wender et al (PH Wender, SS Kety, FS Schulsinger, unpublished data) is presented in Table 3.2. There were 19 suicides in the relatives as a whole, 15 of which were in the biological parents, siblings, and half-siblings of the depressed adoptees. The highly significant concentration of suicide found in both studies occurred in people who were related only genetically to adoptees who had commited suicide or suffered from depression. They did not rear them, were not reared with them, and did not live in the same family environment. In almost all

Table 3.1. Incidence of Suicide in the Relatives* of Adoptees Who Committed Suicide, and Their Controls†

Adoptees	Biological Relatives	Adoptive Relatives
57 adoptees who died by suicide	$\frac{12}{269}$ (4.5%)	$\frac{0}{148}$ (0%)
57 matched control adoptees	$\frac{2}{269}$ (0.7%)	$\frac{0}{150}$ (0%)
	$p < 0.01‡$	

* All identified relatives.
† From Schulsinger F, Kety SS, Rosenthal D, Wender PH: A family study of suicide. In Schou M. Stromgren E (eds): *Origin, Prevention and Treatment of Affective Disorders*. New York, Academic Press, 1979.
‡ Fischer's exact, one-tailed, on Tables 3.1, 3.2, and 3.3.

Table 3.2. Incidence of Suicide in the Relatives of Adoptees Who Have Suffered a Depressive Illness, and Their Controls*

Adoptees	Biological Relatives	Adoptive Relatives
71 adoptees with depression	$\frac{15}{407}$ (3.7%)	$\frac{1}{187}$ (0.5%)
71 matched control adoptees	$\frac{1}{360}$ (0.3%)	$\frac{2}{171}$ (1.2%)
	$p < 0.01$	

* From PH Wender, SS Kety, FS Schulsinger, unpublished data.

cases, the biological relatives were unaware of the whereabouts of the adoptee or what had happened to him.

One would not, of course, conclude from such results that suicide is entirely a genetically determined pattern of behavior in the face of the vast literature which supports the operation of a number of crucial environmental factors. It is more likely that of all individuals who are subjected to some stressful life process or event, those who commit suicide have a genetic predisposition to do so. That raises the question: What may that predisposition be?

Elsewhere in this volume will be found the accumulating evidence from analyses of blood, cerebrospinal fluid, and postmortem brain samples, for metabolites of serotonin or measurement of its receptors, which suggest that some deficiency in serotonin activity somewhere within the brain may be associated with suicide (see Chapter 4).

Among these studies an especially interesting one was carried out on a group of normal volunteers (9). Blood samples were analyzed for platelet monoamine oxidase, and a questionnaire about the individual's family and his patterns of behavior was completed. The groups with the highest and lowest levels of monoamine oxidase were then compared with respect to their answers to the questionnaires. Among a number of findings, the most interesting one pertinent to this discussion is that those students with the lowest levels of this enzyme in their platelets had 8 times the prevalence of suicide in their families compared to the students with high levels of the enzyme. Such results certainly suggest that serotonin metabolism may have some role in suicide, possibly in the expression of the genetic factors involved, since monoamine oxidase is an important enzyme in the further metabolism and inactivation of serotonin.

We can also ask: What is the behavioral trait which is genetically transmitted? Is it depression itself which sometimes leads directly to suicide? This, of course, would be an easy conclusion to draw since there is such a high incidence of suicide in depression and also of depression preceeding suicide. Eli Robins (10), who studied 134 suicides exhaustively, found that a diagnosis of clinical depression could be made in the majority of such individuals. It has been pointed out, however, (11) that whereas 62% of those over 60 years of age were diagnosed in that series with affective disorder, that was true for only 24% of those under 40 years. Instead, in the latter age group, 54% had histories which could be interpreted as showing violence or impulsivity.

If the incidence of suicide in the biological relatives of depressed adoptees is broken down according to the type of affective disorder diagnosed in the adoptee (Table 3.3), it can be seen that whether the adoptees' diagnoses were affect reaction, neurotic depression, bipolar or unipolar depression, there was a significant concentration of suicide in the biological relatives of each group. It is also interesting that the very

Table 3.3. Incidence of Suicide in the Biological Relatives of Depressive and Control Adoptees

Diagnosis in Adoptee	Incidence of Suicide in Biological Relatives	p
Affective reaction	$\frac{5}{66}$ (7.6%)	0.0004*
Neurotic depression	$\frac{3}{127}$ (2.4%)	0.056
Bipolar depression	$\frac{4}{75}$ (5.3%)	0.0036
Unipolar depression	$\frac{3}{139}$ (2.2%)	0.067
No mental illness	$\frac{1}{360}$ (0.3%)	

*Compared with biological relatives of control adoptees with no known history of mental illness.

highest incidence of suicide was in the biological relatives of the adoptees with the very transient syndrome which in Denmark was called "affect reaction." This is usually initiated by a serious suicide attempt followed by a depression of very brief duration with no known recurrence. These individuals did not come back into the psychiatric register. It was apparently an impulsive act almost always precipitated by some stressful life event. There was more than 3 times the prevalence of suicide in the biological relatives of these adoptees than in those of the unipolar depressions, which would be the paradigm of severe chronic depressive illness.

Roy (12) and Tsuang (13) simultaneously and independently found significantly higher risk for suicidal behavior in the families of patients who committed suicide than in the relatives of those who did not. Thus, there appears to be a genetic factor favoring suicide which may operate independently of, or additively with, depression or other major psychosis. It is an interesting possibility that the genetic predisposition to suicide may represent a tendency to impulsive behavior of which suicide is a prime example. There have been a number of studies compatible with that suggestion. Brown and his associates (14) found diminished levels of 5-hydroxyindoleacetic acid in the cerebrospinal fluid of individuals who were not depressed but who were characterized by impulsive or sociopathic behavior. Lithium, which is often effective in the prophylaxis of depression, has also been found to be effective in impulsive and aggressive behavior (15). It would be difficult to find out in a controlled manner, but interesting to know, whether antidepressant drugs or precursors which act primarily to enhance the activity of serotonin in the brain are capable of suppressing suicidal tendencies specifically.

We cannot dismiss the possibility that the genetic factor in suicide is an inability to control impulsive behavior, while depression and other mental illness as well as overwhelming environmental stress serve as potentiating mechanisms which foster or trigger the impulsive behavior, directing it toward a suicidal outcome. In any case, suicide illustrates better than any of the mental illnesses which are more difficult to define and ascertain the very crucial and important interactions between genetic factors and environmental influences.

References

1. Dublin L: *Suicide: A Sociological and Statistical Study.* New York, Ronald Press, 1963.
2. Tsuang MT: Suicide in schizophrenia, manics, depressives, and surgical controls: a comparison with general population suicide mortality. *Arch Gen Psychiatry* 35:153–155, 1978.
3. Roy A: Risk factors for suicide in psychiatric patients. *Arch Gen Psychiatry* 39:1089–1095, 1982.
4. Kallmann F, Anastasio M: Twin studies on the psychopathology of suicide. *J Nerv Ment Dis* 105:40–55, 1947.
5. Haberlandt W: Aportacion a la genetica del suicidio. *Folio Clin Int* 17:319–322, 1967.
6. Juel-Nielson N, Videbech T: A twin study of suicide. *Acta Genet Med Gemellol* 19:307–310, 1970.
7. Kety SS, Rosenthal D, Wender PH, Schulsinger F: The types and prevalence of mental illness in the biological and adoptive families of adopted schizophrenics. In Rosenthal D, Kety SS, (eds): *The Transmission of Schizophrenia.* Oxford, Pergamon Press, 1968.
8. Schulsinger F, Kety SS, Rosenthal D, Wender PH: A family study of suicide. In Schou M, Stromgren E, (eds): *Origin, Prevention and Treatment of Affective Disorders.* New York, Academic Press, 1979.
9. Buchsbaum MS, Coursey RD, Murphy DI: The biochemical high-risk paradigm: behavioral and familial correlates of low platelet monoamine oxidase activity. *Science* 194:339–341, 1976.
10. Robins E: *The Final Months: A Study of the Lives of 134 Persons Who Committed Suicide.* New York, Oxford University Press, 1981.
11. Carlson GA: More analysis of Eli Robins' suicide data. *Am J Psychiatry* 141:323, 1984.
12. Roy A: Family history of suicide. *Arch Gen Psychiatry* 40:971–974, 1983.
13. Tsuang MT: Risk of suicide in the relatives of schizophrenics, manics, depressives, and controls. *J Clin Psychiatry* 44:396–400, 1983.
14. Brown GL, Ebert MH, Goyer PF, Jimerson DC, Klein WJ, Bunny WE, Goodwin FK: Aggression, suicide and serotonin: relationship to CSF amine metabolism. *Am J Psychiatry* 139:741–746, 1982.
15. Shard M, Marini J, Bridges C, Wagner E: The effect of lithium on impulsive, aggressive behavior in man. *Am J Psychiatry* 133:1409–1413, 1976.

4

Biological Factors in Suicide

Marie Åsberg, M.D., Peter Nordström, M.D., and Lil Träskman-Bendz, M.D.

Modern research on suicide has largely been focused on the role of psychological and social problems as causes of self-destructive behavior. Biological factors have rarely been considered of any importance. In a bibliography (1) of research on suicide published between 1958 and 1967, only five of 1267 titles deal with biological subjects. Suicide is generally conceived of as an exclusively human behavior, which presupposes intentionality and a concept of death, and whose biological background, if any, is remote and irrelevant.

Recently, however, two lines of study have suggested that suicidal behavior may indeed have biological correlates, within and possibly also outside the depressive disorders. Two clusters of biological factors have emerged that tend to correlate with suicidal behavior—namely, variables associated with serotonergic neurotransmission and variables associated with certain neuroendocrine functions, particularly the release of cortisol and thyrotropin.

The evidence of biological involvement in some cases of suicide will be reviewed in this chapter. Since most of it emanates from research on the psychobiology of depression, a brief review will be given of current thinking and some methodological issues in that field.

MONOAMINES AND DEPRESSIVE DISORDERS

The hypothesis that certain neurotransmitters are important to the development of psychiatric illness dates back to 1954. Impressed with the chemical similarity between the putative transmitter serotonin and certain hallucinogenic drugs (e.g., lysergic acid diethylamide), Woolley and Shaw (2) suggested that schizophrenia might be caused by abnormal serotonin transmission.

During the 1960s it was realized that administration of reserpine, which depletes brain stores of serotonin, noradrenaline, and dopamine, could cause severe depression of the melancholic type. Reserpine is obtained from *Rauwolfia serpentina*, a plant which had long been used in Indian medicine to sedate psychotic patients. Reserpine reduces blood pressure and was used in western medicine for this purpose, but its use has been largely abandoned because of the depressive symptoms that develop during treatment in about 15% of the patients.

Meanwhile, pharmacologists discovered that antidepressant drugs, both the monoamine oxidase inhibitors and the tricyclic compounds of the imipramine type, also interfere with the turnover of the monoamines in the central nervous system. The monoamine oxidase inhibitors block a pathway for metabolic degradation of mono-amines, while the tricyclic antidepressants block the neuronal reuptake of noradrena-line and/or serotonin, limiting their access to the degradating enzyme.

These insights led to the formulation of two hypotheses relating depression to biochemical disturbances—namely, the noradrenaline hypothesis (3) and the serotonin hypothesis (4). Both hypotheses assert relationships between depression and a reduced amount of the transmitter at certain neuronal receptors in the central nervous system.

Although later research has shown that the early concepts of antidepressant drug action were oversimplified, the noradrenaline and the serotonin hypotheses have been of great heuristic value. In attempts at providing hard evidence of an association between monoamine neurotransmission and depression, concentrations have been measured of the transmitters, their metabolites, and the amino acids used for their synthesis. The activity of enzymes involved in their degradation and the number and affinity characteristics of the tissue components to which they are bound have been studied. Since it is not yet possible to make such measurements in the living human brain, indirect methods have been developed, such as autopsy studies, spinal fluid studies, and studies in which blood platelets serve as models for neurons.

Monoamines in the Brain

Studies of monoamines and monoamine metabolites in brains from people who had committed suicide began to be published in the mid-1960s. It was then often assumed that the majority of the suicide victims were depressed prior to death, and that studies of suicide would yield information about depression, and to some extent this is true. About half of those who commit suicide are retrospectively diagnosed as having suffered from a depressive *syndrome*, while the majority of suicide victims have had depressive *symptoms* prior to death (5).

There are difficult methodological problems in the interpretation of the autopsy studies. The time and mode of death, previous drug treatment, and decay of the amines or their metabolites between death and discovery of the body, and subsequent autopsy, are all important factors and difficult to ascertain. These problems have been widely discussed, e.g., by Beskow and co-workers (6), who failed to find any differences in concentrations of serotonin or its metabolite, 5-hydroxyindoleacetic acid (5-HIAA) between suicide victims and controls, once correction was made for the postmortem delay in the suicide victims.

Table 4.1 summarizes some controlled studies of monoamines and their metabolites in brains from suicide victims. In most of these studies, suicide victims have lower concentrations of serotonin in certain parts of the brain. There is a relatively pro-nounced circadian variation in serotonin concentrations in brain, particularly in the hypothalamus (7). This might lead to erroneous conclusions about group differences, if clock-time of death varies between the groups. Clock-time of death was accounted for, however, in the study by Korpi et al (8), where lower serotonin concentrations were found in the hypothalamus in suicide victims.

The study by Lloyd and co-workers (9) is interesting, despite the small number of subjects. Lloyd et al measured serotonin concentrations, not in large sections of the brain as previous researchers had done, but in discrete nuclei in the raphe region of the brainstem, where the cell bodies of most of the serotonin neurons in the brain are located. The suicide victims were found to have significantly lower serotonin concen-trations in some of the raphe nuclei studied, but not in all. The lowest serotonin concentrations were found in the dorsal raphe nucleus, which projects to the limbic system, and the *nucleus centralis inferior*, which projects to the spinal cord.

Table 4.1. Some Controlled Studies of Monoamines and Their Metabolites in Brains from Suicide Victims

Author	Subjects	Analyses	Result
Shaw et al (126)	22 suicides (11 depressed), 17 controls	Serotonin in hindbrain	Suicides < controls
Bourne et al (127)	23 suicides (16 depressed), 28 controls	Serotonin, 5-HIAA, noradrenaline in hindbrain	No difference, except lower 5-HIAA in depressed subjects
Pare et al (128)	26 suicides, 15 controls	Serotonin, noradrenaline, dopamine in brainstem, hypothalamus, caudate	Serotonin: suicides < controls, otherwise no differences
Lloyd et al (9)	7 suicides, 5 controls	Serotonin and 5-HIAA in six raphe nuclei	Serotonin: suicides < controls in nuclei raphe dorsalis and centralis inferior
Cochran et al (129)	10 depressed and 9 alcoholic suicides, 12 controls	Serotonin in several brain areas	No differences between suicides and controls
Beskow et al (6)	23 suicides, 62 controls	Serotonin, noradrenaline, dopamine, 5-HIAA, and HVA in several brain areas	No differences after adjustment for longer postmortem delay in suicides
Korpi et al (8)	29 healthy controls, 30 schizophrenics (50% dead from suicide), 14 nonschizophrenic suicides	Serotonin, tryptophan, and 5-HIAA in several areas	Serotonin in hypothalamus lower in nonschizophrenic suicides

Monoamine Metabolites

A widely used method of obtaining information about the turnover of the monoamines in the brain is to measure their metabolites in cerebrospinal fluid (CSF), usually obtained by lumbar puncture. The metabolite concentrations are in the nanomolar range, and highly sensitive and specific analytical methods are needed to measure them with sufficient accuracy.

There has been some discussion as to whether concentrations of, for example, the serotonin metabolite, 5-HIAA, in CSF reflect serotonin turnover in the spinal cord rather than in the brain itself. The demonstration by Stanley and co-workers (M Stanley, L Träskman-Bendz, K Dorovini-Zis, unpublished data, 1985) that 5-HIAA in CSF drawn after death correlates strongly with 5-HIAA in brain cortex suggests, however, that brain events are indeed reflected in CSF metabolite concentrations.

A main advantage of the CSF technique is that spinal fluid is comparatively easy to obtain at little discomfort to the patient. There are many disadvantages as well. The

Table 4.2. Some Factors of Importance for the Concentration of 5-HIAA Measured in Lumbar Spinal Fluid Samples

Factor	Possible Control Measure
Subject's age and sex*	Matched controls or analysis of co-variance
Subject's body height†	Idem
Physical illness‡	Physically healthy subjects
Drug treatment§	Drug-free subjects
Time of day¶	Samples always drawn at the same time
Time of year‖	Patients and controls matched for season
Diet**	Fasting subjects or controlled diet
Physical movement††	Bed rest prior to lumbar puncture
Subject's position at lumbar puncture‡‡	Same position always used
Intervertebral space used for puncture§§	Same interstitium always used
Amount of CSF drawn¶¶	Same amount always drawn
Handling and storage of samples	Identical procedures for all samples
Analytical method‖‖	Best available method

* See review by Asberg and Bertilsson (130).
† Wode-Helgodt and Sedvall (131); see also Åsberg and Bertilsson (130).
‡ Some physical illnesses are associated with alterations of CSF 5-HIAA, e.g., Parkinson's disease (132), multiple sclerosis (133), adult celiac disease (134), and hydrocephalus (135).
§ Treatment with antidepressant drugs may lower CSF 5-HIAA (13, 136–140).
¶ There is a circadian variation in ventricular CSF 5-HIAA (141).
‖ There is some evidence of a circannual variation in CSF 5-HIAA (23, 142).
** It cannot be excluded that a diet particularly rich (or poor) in monoamine precursors might influence the metabolite concentrations. Thus, underweight anorexia nervosa patients have significantly lower CSF 5-HIAA than recently weight-recovered and long term weight-recovered anorectics (143).
†† Physical exercise raises CSF 5-HIAA (144).
‡‡ There is some preliminary evidence of lower CSF levels if the puncture is performed when the patient lies down (G Sedvall and G Oxentierna, personal communication).
§§ Significantly higher 5-HIAA levels are obtained when the punctures are performed between vertebrae L3 and L4 than between L4 and L5 in the same subject (145).
¶¶ Due to a concentration gradient of 5-HIAA in the lumbar CSF, the concentration increases the more CSF is taken. Spurious differences between patients and controls can then easily be created by drawing unequal amounts of CSF in the two categories (146).
‖‖ Comparisons between the earlier spectrophotofluorometry methods and the more recent mass fragmentography have clearly shown the advantages of the latter (147–149).

concentrations of 5-HIAA and of the dopamine metabolite, homovanillic acid (HVA), depend inter alia on the subject's sex, age, and body height. The dependence on body height is presumably due to an active removal from CSF of the acid metabolites as they flow from the brain ventricles down to the lumbar sac where the CSF is sampled.

Metabolite concentrations also vary seasonally and with the time of the day. Most important in clinical studies, the concentrations are drastically altered by treatment with certain psychotropic drugs. A summary of some factors of importance to the concentration of 5-HIAA in lumbar CSF is given in Table 4.2.

In view of the formidable methodological problems, it will come as no surprise to the reader that the available evidence for altered monoamine metabolite concentrations in CSF in depression is not as conclusive as might be wished. However, a review by Post and co-workers (10) suggests that the average concentration of 5-HIAA in depressed patients is reduced to about 78% of that in controls (average of 15 published studies). Data from a recent study of 83 patients with melancholia and 66 healthy controls bear this out, showing significantly lower concentrations of 5-HIAA and HVA in the depressives after correction for sex, age, and height by analysis of co-variance (11).

In spite of its relatively uniform clinical picture, melancholia may be pathophysiologically heterogeneous. Low concentrations of CSF 5-HIAA are found in only 30% of patients, and in several studies the distributions of the metabolite tend toward bimodality (12–15).

Van Praag and co-workers have suggested that low CSF 5-HIAA may be an indicator of vulnerability to depression. In line with this contention, they have found an increased incidence of depressive illness in *relatives* of patients with low CSF 5-HIAA, as compared with relatives of normal 5-HIAA patients (16). This finding is reminiscent of the observation by Sedvall and co-workers (17) that healthy subjects with a family history of depressive illness had lower CSF 5-HIAA than healthy subjects without such a history. Preliminary data from twin studies by Sedvall and co-workers (18) further support familial implication in CSF concentrations of the monoamine metabolites.

A vulnerability or "trait" marker would be expected to remain fairly constant over prolonged periods. However, most serotonin-related variables seem to vary seasonally. Seasonal rhythms have been shown for the serotonin concentration in human hypothalamus (7), for the platelet serotonin uptake (19, 20; R Malmgren, A Åberg-Wistedt, B Mårtensson, M Åsberg, unpublished data, 1984), and for the platelet [³H]imipramine binding (21, 22). There is some evidence that a seasonal rhythm, very similar to that observed for serotonin in hypothalamus, may exist also for CSF 5-HIAA (23). Seasonal rhythm is a complicating factor where stability over time is under consideration.

The bulk of the evidence suggests that 5-HIAA concentrations in CSF remain fairly stable over limited periods in normal subjects, and in depressed patients readmitted for relapse of depression (24). Recovered depressives, whose 5-HIAA concentrations are normal during illness, also remain stable over prolonged periods, whereas in depressives with low 5-HIAA during illness the concentration sometimes increases with recovery but remains in the low range in most cases. The relevant studies are summarized in Table 4.3.

It should be pointed out that CSF studies of recovered depressives are necessarily rare. Such patients are often maintained on drugs for extended periods, and those who are not, even if available for lumbar puncture studies, may well be nonrepresentative of the majority of the depressed population.

A possible interpretation of the existing data is that there is a subgroup of depressed patients, characterized by concentrations of CSF 5-HIAA that are not only low but also less stable over time. If this type of unstable serotonin system is associated with an increased vulnerability to illness, and with a further decrease in release during illness, the emergence of bimodal distributions in diseased populations is easily explained.

Table 4.3. Changes in CSF 5-HIAA after Recovery from Depression

Author	Type of 5-HIAA Measure	No.	Time Lag	Results
Coppen et al (150)	Baseline 5-HIAA	8	3–59 weeks	Stable over time
van Praag (151)	Probenecid-induced accumulation of 5-HIAA	50	> 6 months	< 50% of patients with low CSF 5-HIAA during illness normalized; the rest remained stable
Post et al (10)	5-HIAA after probenecid	11	Several months	Stable over time
Träskman-Bendz et al (24)	Baseline 5-HIAA	11	2–7 years	Increased concentrations at follow-up in patients whose levels were low during illness; stable in the remainder

In contrast to central serotonin and 5-HIAA, the release of noradrenaline in the central nervous system is thought to be mirrored in urinary concentrations of the noradrenaline metabolite, 3-methoxy-4-hydroxyphenyl glycol (MHPG). Urinary 5-HIAA is probably derived to a very large extent from the gastrointestinal tract, whereas a substantial proportion of the urinary MHPG is thought to emanate from the brain. Urinary concentrations of MHPG have therefore been measured extensively in the depressive disorders, and there is relatively good agreement that they are reduced, particularly in the bipolar type of depression (25–27). CSF concentrations of the noradrenaline metabolite, MHPG, are apparently normal in depressive illness (11).

Precursors

The rate-limiting enzyme for serotonin synthesis, tryptophan hydroxylase, is not fully saturated at physiological precursor concentrations. This means that the amount of serotonin in brain is regulated by the amount of the precursor amino acid, tryptophan, that is available for its synthesis. The availability is a function of the plasma concentration of tryptophan and of its transport into the central nervous system. Since several amino acids compete for the same carrier system, the ratio of tryptophan to other neutral amino acids will be the important factor (28).

There is some evidence that plasma concentrations of free tryptophan are low in melancholic depression, although there are also conflicting findings (see review, 29). The ratio of plasma tryptophan to other neutral amino acids was decreased in two studies of depressed patients (30, 31), and appeared to predict the effect of tryptophan treatment in another study (32). The finding is particularly interesting in view of the varying results with precursor treatment in depressive disorder.

Platelet Monoamine Oxidase (MAO)

In certain ways, blood platelets resemble serotonin neurons: they have an active uptake mechanism for the transmitter; they can store serotonin in special granules; their mitochondria contain MAO which metabolizes the transmitter; and they have binding sites for drugs that block the uptake of serotonin (e.g., imipramine). Since blood platelets are easily accessible, these properties have been widely studied in psychiatric patients, and to some extent in healthy people. It should be borne in mind, when interpreting such studies, that there is yet very little empirical support for a quantitative parellellism between neurons and platelets in these respects.

There is no strong evidence for an alteration of platelet MAO activity in depressive disorder. On the other hand, quite suggestive evidence exists that platelet MAO activity is associated with certain personality traits such as impulsivity and sensation seeking, which may in their turn predispose the individual to some types of psychopathology (33–35).

Platelet MAO activity is genetically regulated, and weakly but consistently related to CSF 5-HIAA (36, 37). Oreland and Shaskan (38) suggested that platelet MAO activity in man may reflect some innate characteristic of the serotonin system, such as its size or capacity, rather than its activity at a given time. This would be in analogy to the number of dopamine neurons in mouse brain, which is reflected in the brain activity of the catecholamine-synthesizing enzyme, tyrosine hydroxylase.

[3H]Imipramine-Binding Sites

An interesting development is the possibility of measuring characteristics of the specific binding of certain drugs to nervous tissue, and to blood platelets which again serve as models for serotonin neurons. The most widely studied binding has been that of tritiated imipramine. The imipramine-binding site is probably presynaptic and is believed to be closely related to (but not identical with) the serotonin uptake site. The endogenous ligand (if any exists) to the imipramine-binding site is not known.

There is fairly good agreement that the number of [3H]imipramine-binding sites on platelet membranes is reduced in depressive disorder (39–41). Perry et al (42) also report a reduced number of imipramine-binding sites in brain from depressives who died a natural death.

Serotonin Uptake

The active *uptake of serotonin* into platelets from depressed patients is reduced (43–47). The difference becomes particularly pronounced when patients and controls are matched for month of blood sampling (R Malmgren, A Åberg-Wistedt, B Mårtensson, M Asberg, unpublished data, 1984). Like CSF 5-HIAA and serotonin concentrations in the hypothalamus, platelet serotonin uptake appears to vary seasonally (20). A serotonin-mediated function, possibly related to the platelet uptake, is the *formation of cyclic guanosine monophosphate* (cGMP) induced by the transmitter. Serotonin-stimulated cGMP formation is inhibited by drugs which block serotonin uptake. Preliminary findings (ML Tjörnhammar, B Mårtensson, M Åsberg, T Bartfai, unpublished data, 1984) suggest that the cGMP formation stimulated by serotonin is much lower in platelets from depressed patients than in control subjects.

Interrelations between "Serotonin Markers"

So far, there is little knowledge of the interrelations between the potential markers of serotonin function, in the healthy person and in disease states. There is an obvious interest in clarifying these relationships, both with a view to understanding their physiological significance and for practical diagnostic purposes.

Interestingly, there are no clear-cut relationships between imipramine binding and serotonin uptake in depressed patients (48). These two possible serotonin markers may thus reflect different aspects of serotonin functions. There is, on the other hand, a significant but relatively weak correlation between CSF 5-HIAA and platelet MAO activity, although only in healthy subjects and not in any of the patient groups studied.

SUICIDE AND SEROTONIN
Low CSF 5-HIAA and Attempted Suicide in Depression

In their attempts to find clinical correlates to a low concentration of CSF 5-HIAA in depressed patients, Åsberg and co-workers (49) unexpectedly found an increased incidence of suicide attempts in the low 5-HIAA subgroup. Forty percent of the low 5-HIAA patients had attempted suicide during their present illness, as compared with 15% in the normal 5-HIAA patients. Furthermore, the attempts were of a more determined nature with a preference for active, violent methods in the low 5-HIAA patients, while those in the high 5-HIAA group were confined to drug overdoses. Two deaths from suicide occurred during the study period, both in low 5-HIAA patients.

The relationship between CSF 5-HIAA and suicidal behavior was confirmed by Ågren (50). He studied depressed patients and measured suicidal behavior by means of the Schedule for Affective Disorder and Schizophrenia (SADS) scales for suicidal behavior. These scales do not differentiate between suicidal ideation and suicidal acts, which may have weakened the correlation. In the Åsberg et al (49) study, there was no association between low CSF 5-HIAA and suicidal ideation, or rated suicide risk.

These early studies did not take into account the relationship between CSF 5-HIAA and such interference factors as sex and body height. Men tend to have a lower CSF 5-HIAA concentration than women, and they are also more prone to use violent methods if they attempt suicide. The sex factor could, however, be ruled out in a subsequent confirmatory study by Träskman et al (51).

More recently, the relationship has been confirmed in Dutch depressed patients studied by van Praag (52), who found a very highly significant increase in suicidal behavior in patients with low probenecid-induced accumulation of 5-HIAA. Lower 5-HIAA concentrations in suicidal than in nonsuicidal depressed patients were also reported by Montgomery and Montgomery (53) in British patients. Palanappian and co-workers (54) found a significant correlation between suicidal tendencies (estimated by the item Suicide in the Hamilton Rating Scale) and CSF 5-HIAA concentrations in Indian depressed patients. Banki and co-workers (55) demonstrated a relationship between low CSF 5-HIAA and suicide attempts in Hungarian female patients. In Banki's study, the association was confined to those who had used active methods. Pérez de los Cobos et al (56) have reported a relationship between suicide attempts and low CSF 5-HIAA in Spanish patients, regardless of the method used in the attempt.

There is also one well designed, nonconfirmatory study by Roy-Byrne and co-workers (57), who mainly studied treatment-resistant American patients, referred to a research center specializing in the study of depressive disorders. No significant relationship was found between lifetime suicidal behavior and CSF 5-HIAA, possibly owing to the high proportion of bipolar (manic-depressive) patients in the group. When their unipolar cases were examined separately, the suicidal unipolars tended to have lower CSF 5-HIAA than other unipolars. The biological correlates of suicidal behavior may thus differ in bipolar and unipolar disorder. A similar conclusion was reached by Ågren (58). The studies are summarized in Table 4.4.

Table 4.4. Studies of CSF 5-HIAA in Relation to Suicidal Behavior

Author	Subjects	Measure of Suicidality	Result
Åsberg et al (49)	68 hospitalized depressed patients	Attempted or completed suicide within index illness episode	Low 5-HIAA in the 15 attempters, particularly those using violent methods
Brown et al (86)	22 men with personality disorder	Lifetime history of suicide attempt	Lower 5-HIAA and higher MHPG in the 11 suicide attempters
Ågren (50)	33 depressed patients	SADS suicidality scale scores	Negative correlations with 5-HIAA and MHPG
Träskman et al (51)	30 suicide attempters (8 depressed, 22 other psychiatric disorders excluding schizophrenia and alcoholism), 45 healthy controls	Recent attempted or completed suicide	5-HIAA lower in attempters than in controls, HVA lower in depressed attempters only
Leckman et al (152)	132 psychiatric patients	Nurses' ratings of suicidal tendencies	Negative correlations with 5-HIAA
Brown et al (59)	12 patients with borderline personality disorder	Lifetime history of suicide	Lower 5-HIAA in the 5 attempters
van Praag (52)	203 depressed patients	Recent suicide attempt	Lower CSF 5-HIAA after probenecid in the 54 suicide attempters
Palanappian et al (54)	40 hospitalized depressed patients	Suicide item in the Hamilton Rating Scale	Negative correlation with CSF 5-HIAA and HVA
Ågren (58)	110 depressed patients	SADS suicidality scales	Negative correlation to CSF 5-HIAA and MHPG
Roy-Byrne et al (57)	32 bipolar, 13 unipolar patients in different phases of illness	Lifetime history of suicide attempt	No association with 5-HIAA

Table 4.4—*Continued*

Author	Subjects	Measure of Suicidality	Result
van Praag (60)	10 nondepressed schizophrenics who attempted suicide in response to imperative hallucinations, 10 nonsuicidal schizophrenics, 10 controls	Recent suicide attempt	Lower CSF 5-HIAA after probenecid in suicide attempters
Banki et al (55)	141 female inpatients (36 depressed, 46 schizoprenic, 35 alcoholic, 24 with adjustment disorder; 45 previously reported)	Recent suicide attempt	Negative correlation with 5-HIAA in all diagnostic groups, particulary with violent attempts; inconsistent relationships to HVA
Ninan et al (61)	8 suicidal, 8 nonsuicidal schizophrenic patients, matched for age and sex	Lifetime history of suicide attempt	Lower 5-HIAA in suicidal patients
Pérez de los Cobos et al (56)	21 depressed patients	Suicide attempt, suicidal ideation rated on the Hamilton Scale and the AMDP system	More attempts and higher suicidality scores in patients with low 5-HIAA

Low CSF 5-HIAA and Suicide Attempts in Other Disorders

As mentioned previously, only about 50% of those who commit suicide are retrospectively diagnosed as having suffered from a depressive syndrome. Several groups have studied the relationship between suicidal behavior and CSF 5-HIAA in other diagnostic categories. Träskman et al (51) found low CSF 5-HIAA in comparison with normals also in *nondepressed* suicide attempters (mainly patients with personality disorders and minor affective disorders). Brown et al (59) studied two groups of men with *personality disorders* and found more lifetime suicidal behavior in those with low CSF 5-HIAA.

Van Praag (60) and Ninan and co-workers (61) found a similar association in *schizophrenia*. Both studies are well designed with carefully chosen, matched controls. Lower CSF 5-HIAA in suicidal patients among subjects with schizophrenia has also been reported by Banki et al (55).

Banki and co-workers (55) have also found a similar relationship in *alcoholism* and *adjustment disorder*. The relationship between low CSF 5-HIAA and suicide attempts thus appears to be surprisingly robust.

The CSF studies summarized above all concerned survivors of a suicide attempt. In a study by Kauert et al (62), suboccipital CSF concentrations of the monoamines serotonin, adrenaline, noradrenaline, and dopamine were measured after death by suicide. Serotonin levels were *increased* in the suicide victims. It cannot be excluded, however, that this unexpected difference may reflect differences in the time of death in suicides and controls. In monkeys, CSF serotonin concentrations are almost doubled during the night, and the daytime mean concentration is only 5% of the peak concentration at nighttime (63).

CSF 5-HIAA as a Predictor of Suicide

Those who attempt and those who commit suicide are well known to differ in many important respects, even if there is an overlap between the two populations (64). In several studies, subsequent mortality from suicide among suicide attempters has amountd to about 2% within a year after the attempt (65). Although this is a considerable increase in suicide frequency over the general population, suicide is a rare event even in this group.

Estimating suicide risk and taking appropriate precautions is one of the most difficult tasks of the practicing psychiatrist. It is therefore of clinical interest to increase the precision of risk evaluation, and there have been many attempts to create rating scales and inventories for the purpose. These have not usually been very successful (66). Could the measurement of CSF 5-HIAA be of any help?

The data presented in Table 4.5 suggest that it might. Among patients who have made a suicide attempt, those with low CSF 5-HIAA are 10 times more likely to die from suicide than the remainder. A similar increase in suicide mortality after a suicide attempt in patients who had low CSF 5-HIAA was found by Roy and co-workers (A Roy, H Ågren, D Pickar, M Linnoila, A Doran, N Cutler, SM Paul, unpublished data, 1985).

On the whole, CSF 5-HIAA concentrations tend to remain similar from one illness episode to another. The authors have, however, made repeated punctures in two patients who subsequently committed suicide. In both cases, there was a substantial *reduction* in CSF 5-HIAA from one puncture to the next. Taken together with the finding that in patients whose CSF 5-HIAA is low during illness, its concentration

Table 4.5. Mortality from Suicide within 1 Year after Admission to Hospital in Some High Risk Groups

Patient Category	No.	Suicides (%)
Patients admitted to intensive care unit after suicide attempt	45	2
Patients admitted to a psychiatric clinic after a suicide attempt, CSF 5-HIAA above 90 nmoles/liter	42	2
Patients admitted to a psychiatric clinic after a suicide attempt, CSF 5-HIAA below 90 nmoles/liter	34	21

increases on recovery, the observation suggests that failure to maintain a stable serotonin transmission may be of pathophysiological significance.

MAO in Brain and Platelets

The activity of MAO in brain regions from suicide victims was similar to that of controls in two studies (67, 68). Gottfries et al (69), however, found a lower MAO activity in alcoholic suicide victims than in controls.

There is some evidence that platelet MAO activity is related to suicidal behavior. Buchsbaum and co-workers (70) found an increased frequency of psychosocial problems, including suicide attempts in college students with very low activity of platelet MAO. Among the relatives of these students, the incidence of suicide attempts was significantly higher than among high MAO probands.

Studies of platelet MAO activity in suicidal psychiatric patients have been few and the results not unequivocal. Buchsbaum and co-workers (71) found a relationship between low platelet MAO and suicide in psychiatric patients, but only if they were also augmenters in averaged evoked response tests. Gottfries and co-workers (72) reported that depressed patients who had made violent suicide attempts had significantly lower platelet MAO activity than other depressives, including those who had taken drug overdoses.

Binding Studies in Suicide Victims

The development of methods for studying the specific binding of drugs to brain tissue has reawakened interest in autopsy studies of suicide victims. So far, the most intensively studied ligand has been [^{3}H]imipramine. Stanley and co-workers (73) and Paul and co-workers (73a) found lower imipramine binding in suicide victims. In contrast, Meyerson and co-workers (74) report *increased* imipramine binding in suicide victims as compared with controls.

The imipramine-binding site is probably related to the presynaptic serotonin uptake site. Stanley and Mann (75) also measured postsynaptic, serotonin-2-binding sites with [^{3}H]spiroperidol in their suicide cases. In agreement with a hypothesis of reduced serotonin release in suicidal patients, they found an increased number of binding sites. The correlation between imipramine and spiroperidol binding was negative although nonsignificant, possibly due to the small number of subjects. A nonsignificant increase in serotonin-2 binding was also reported by Owen et al (76).

Muscarinic binding of [^{3}H]quinuclidinyl benzilate (QNB) was normal in the suicide victims studied by Stanley (77) and by Kaufmann and co-workers (78). In contrast, the Meyerson et al (74) study quoted above reports an increased QNB binding in suicide victims.

5-Hydroxytryptophan-Induced Cortisol Release

Meltzer and co-workers (79, 80) made a very interesting attempt to study serotonin functions beyond the postsynaptic receptor. They measured the response in blood cortisol concentration to infusions of the serotonin precursor, 5-hydroxytryptophan. Normally, this procedure leads to a slight increase in serum cortisol. The cortisol release is much exaggerated in depressive illness. When the depressed patients were subdivided into those who had made suicide attempts, those who had suicidal thoughts, and those who were nonsuicidal, the cortisol reaction was clearly enhanced in the attempters. This finding is in line with the hypothesis of a reduced release of serotonin in suicide attempters, which would tend to cause hypersensitivity of serotonin receptors. It also provides an interesting correlation to the cluster of endocrine variables that also correlate with suicide.

Melatonin and Magnesium

Recently two studies have appeared where two other biological variables, melatonin in plasma and magnesium in CSF, have been related to suicidal behavior. Since both are in certain respects related to serotonin, they will be discussed here.

Beck-Friis and co-workers (81) reported that the nocturnal serum melatonin concentrations known to be decreased in depression (82, 82a) were closer to normal in suicidal than in nonsuicidal patients. Melatonin production is influenced by light and thought to be regulated by β-adrenergic neurotransmission. Serotonin is a precursor of melatonin, although little is known of any correlation between the concentrations of the two compounds in man.

Banki and co-workers (83) found a relationship between low CSF concentrations of magnesium and suicide attempts. There was a strong positive correlation between CSF magnesium and CSF 5-HIAA. Interestingly, melatonin concentrations in CSF are strongly correlated to CSF magnesium concentrations (83a).

SUICIDE AND OTHER MONOAMINES
Dopamine

The concentrations of the dopamine metabolite, HVA, in CSF are reduced in depression (10), and more consistently so than CSF 5-HIAA, to which they are strongly correlated. Whether the correlation between the two metabolites is due to their sharing the same transport mechanism or to a functional connection between the parent amines is not known.

Low concentrations of HVA in suicidal depressed patients have been reported by Träskman et al (51), by Montgomery and Montgomery (53), and by Ågren (58). In the follow-up of depressed patients by Roy et al (A Roy, H Ågren, D Pickar, M Linnoila, A Doran, N Cutler, SM Paul, unpublished data, 1985), a low level of HVA was an even better predictor of subsequent suicide than was 5-HIAA.

Banki et al (55) found a less clear-cut relationship between suicide and HVA than with 5-HIAA. In particular, their depressed patients who had taken drug overdoses had significantly higher HVA than nonsuicidal patients, while HVA in violent attempters was very low. In the Träskman et al study, only the suicide attempters who were also depressed had lower than normal HVA concentrations. This may suggest that the reduced HVA concentrations may be more closely related to some particular aspect of depressive illness than to suicidal behavior in general. Only depressive suicide attempters were included in the studies of Montgomery and Montgomery, Ågren, and Roy et al. The failure of Ninan et al (84) to find any difference in CSF HVA between their suicidal and nonsuicidal schizophrenic subjects is in line with this.

Noradrenaline

In comparison with the evidence relating suicide to serotonin, the relationships with noradrenaline are less clear. Ågren (85) reported a negative correlation between the noradrenaline metabolite, MHPG, and suicidal tendencies in their depressed patients. Brown and co-workers (86) found a positive correlation in subjects with personality disorders which was not reproduced in their study (59) of borderline patients. Ostroff and associates measured the ratio between noradrenaline and adrenaline in urine in two studies (87, 88) of mixed diagnostic groups and found a relationship between a low ratio and suicidal behavior.

NEUROENDOCRINOLOGY AND SUICIDE

Over recent years, a series of psychoendocrine disturbances has been described in the depressive disorders. The most extensively documented ones are a blunted thyrotropin response (TSH) to the injection of thyrotropin-releasing hormone (TRH), and an activation of the hypothalamic-pituitary-adrenal axis (evidenced by high cortisol levels in blood, urine, and CSF, a disturbance of their circadian and circannual rhythms, and an inability to suppress cortisol release after administration of such synthetic corticosteroids as dexamethasone). Reviews of the two areas of research have been published by Loosen and Prange (89) and Carroll (90).

There is fairly good agreement among investigators that the dexamethasone suppression test (DST) is abnormal in about 60% of patients with the melancholic subtype of major depressive disorder. There is less agreement as to whether the disturbances are specific for melancholia, although this has been strongly claimed, for example by Carroll (90). However, abnormal DSTs have also been reported in demented, schizophrenic, and alcoholic patients, in anxiety states, and in obsessive-compulsive disorder.

An abnormal DST is very likely to be state-dependent, since it normalizes with recovery from depression.

Blunted TRH/TSH responses are seen in 25 to 50% of patients with depressive disorders and in occasional alcoholic patients (even when they have been abstinent for years). Most studies report no relationship between the DST and the TRH/TSH tests (91).

Other endocrine abnormalities (e.g., disturbance of the release of growth hormone) have been described in depression, but since they have not yet been specifically associated with suicide they will not be discussed here.

Suicide and the Hypothalamic-Pituitary-Adrenal Axis

In 1965, Bunney and Fawcett (92) reported that patients who went on to seriously attempt or to complete suicide had an unusually high excretion of cortisol metabolites prior to the event. In 1969, Bunney and co-workers (93) replicated the findings and suggested that the measurement of cortisol might be useful in identifying people at risk for suicide. Although there has been some doubt as to the usefulness of the test for measuring suicide potential (94), and it does not seem to have been widely used, very similar findings were made by Ostroff and colleagues in 1982 (87).

In a prospective study, Krieger (95) demonstrated a relationship between high cortisol concentrations in blood and ultimate suicide. Träskman and co-workers (96) found high CSF concentrations of cortisol in suicidal patients, but only in those who were depressed as well. Banki and co-workers (55) found no relationship between CSF cortisol and suicidal tendencies in any of the diagnostic categories studied, which agrees with the normal concentrations of cortisol in brains from suicide victims, studied by Brooksbank and co-workers (97).

The introduction of the DST has renewed interest in the suicide-cortisol association. Carroll and co-workers (98) found abnormal DSTs more often in suicidal than in nonsuicidal patients, but the relationship was confined to patients with melancholia. Agren (50) found no relationship between an abnormal DST and suicidal behavior measured by the SADS scales, but Coryell and Schlesser (99) and Targum and co-workers (100) did find a relationship in depressed patients. Robbins and Alessi (101) found a similar relationship in adolescents, most of whom were also depressed. Banki and co-workers (55) also found a relationship between abnormal DST and suicidality, but in their case also in schizophrenics, alcoholics, and patients with adjustment disorder (but the frequency of abnormal DSTs was unusually high in all of these categories).

Suicide and the Thyroid Axis

The blunted TSH response to TRH seen in depression has been associated both with an increased incidence of suicide attempts and of completed suicide, as reported by Linkowski and co-workers (102, 103). In contrast to their findings, Banki and associates (55) reported a *higher* TSH response to TRH in suicidal than in nonsuicidal psychiatric patients. The reason for the discrepancy is not known, but it is interesting to note that Ågren (85) found that baseline plasma TSH correlated in different directions with different suicide scales from the SADS.

INTERRELATIONS BETWEEN MONOAMINES AND ENDOCRINE VARIABLES

Monoaminergic neurons are known to be involved in the chain of events that leads to release of many hormones, including cortisol. The details of this have not yet been worked out, but the data from the Meltzer et al (79, 80) study of 5-hydroxytryptophan-induced release of cortisol strongly suggest a functional connection between the serotonin system and the hypothalamic-pituitary-adrenal (HPA) axis.

The available data in man do not, however, show any negative correlations between markers of the systems, such as might be expected if they reflect an identical risk factor for suicide. Thus CSF concentrations of cortisol and of 5-HIAA have been shown to correlate positively, though weakly (96) or not at all (82; A-K Aminoff, M Åsberg, L Bertilsson, P Eneroth, B Mårtensson, L Träskman-Bendz, unpublished data, 1985). Carroll et al (104) and Banki and Arató (105) found a positive correlation between postdexamethasone cortisol and 5-HIAA. The interpretation of the results from Carroll et al is, however, complicated by the fact that spinal fluid was drawn after the administration of dexamethasone, which raises CSF 5-HIAA concentrations (105a).

Among other potential markers of serotonin, the ratio of *l*-tryptophan to other neutral amino acids was positively correlated to postdexamethasone cortisol (31), while V_{max} of serotonin uptake into platelets (which is reduced in depression) tended to be negatively correlated to an abnormal DST (106).

Gold and co-workers (107) report an inverse correlation between the magnitude of the TSH reaction to TRH and CSF 5-HIAA. The negative correlation between the TRH/TSH test and CSF 5-HIAA appears also in the study by Banki and co-workers (55), where it is compatible with their finding of more normal TRH/TSH responses in suicidal than in nonsuicidal patients.

TOWARD A PSYCHOBIOLOGY OF SUICIDE?

Apparently, both a low CSF 5-HIAA and an activation of the HPA axis are associated with an increased risk for suicide. The absence of reports of negative correlations between the two markers suggests that they may be independent and associated with suicide through different mechanisms.

Although the nature of these mechanisms is far from clear, the available data do allow some speculation. The HPA activation, for instance, has long been regarded as a consequence of emotional stress and failing defenses (108). Recently, strong support for the stress hypothesis was provided in a study by Ceulemans et al (109), who found almost 50% abnormal DSTs immediately prior to surgery for herniated discs in otherwise healthy, nondepressed individuals. The nonsuppressors had higher scores in inventories for state anxiety, whereas their trait anxiety scores were similar to those of the suppressors, suggesting that anticipatory anxiety prior to surgery was indeed the reason for the HPA activation.

If the HPA activation reflects the emotional suffering and subjective helplessness associated with depressive illness, the relationship with suicide makes intuitive sense. The abnormal DST may function as an alert signal that the emotional pain is approaching unbearable levels.

With a low CSF 5-HIAA, the situation is slightly different. Low 5-HIAA concentrations occur also in mentally healthy people who have never been depressed or contemplated suicide. This has led to the hypothesis that 5-HIAA is a marker of vulnerability.

In most individuals with a low CSF 5-HIAA, vulnerability will never be manifested in a suicide attempt. A suicide attempt is unlikely to occur unless the individual finds himself in a situation which he conceives of as desperate, or when he is without hope for the future. Adverse events may have created this situation, or the individual's perception of the situation may be colored by depressive illness. Whether this state of affairs leads to a suicide attempt is partially determined by the quality of the person's social support net, which may attenuate the effect of adverse events or render the sufferings of depressive illness more tolerable. Previous experience of adverse events (e.g., during childhood) is likely to render the interpretation of current adversity more ominous.

A low output serotonin system (or perhaps even more likely, a low stability one) might render an individual more vulnerable to self-destructive or impulsive action in time of crisis. This characteristic of the serotonin system might have a genetic basis, or it might be acquired. There are suggestions that "learned helplessness" situations in rats may lead to functional changes in the monoamine systems (110) and that prolonged social isolation in mice consistently reduces serotonin turnover (111).

The mice data are particularly interesting, since the magnitude of the reduction is apparently under genetic control. It differs between inbred mice strains and interestingly parallels the strain differences in aggressive behavior released by the isolation.

If serotonin transmission is permanently low or unstable in suicide-prone individuals, it is conceivable that this may be manifested in other ways than in suicidal tendencies. The often quite unpremeditated, impulsive, and violent character of many of the suicide attempts in low 5-HIAA patients suggests that they might have difficulties with impulse control, particularly perhaps in the control of aggressive impulses (49). What, then, is the evidence of a connection between serotonin and aggression in man?

Serotonin and Aggressive Behavior

Early psychoanalytic authors stressed the aggressive component in suicidal behavior and in depressive illness (112). Serotonin neurons are involved in the control of aggressive behavior in animals (111), and treatment with inhibitors of serotonin synthesis may provoke uncontrollable rage in docile domestic cats and make nursing rat mothers bite their young to death (113).

In an investigation of the hypothesis that aggression dyscontrol was the link between serotonin turnover and suicidal behavior, Brown and associates (86) studied men with personality disorders. They were rated for aggression on the basis of lifetime history of overt hostile and destructive behavior. A significant inverse correlation was found between CSF 5-HIAA and overt aggression.

Brown et al (59) gave personality inventories to their subjects in an extended study and found an inverse relationship between CSF 5-HIAA and the Pd scale from the Minnesota Multiphasic Personality Inventory (MMPI). They did not, however, find any significant relationship to self-reported aggressive feelings, as measured by the Buss Durkee Inventory. Rydin and co-workers (114) compared hostility, rated on the basis of Rorschach protocols, in otherwise matched pairs of psychiatric patients with low vis-à-vis high CSF 5-HIAA. Low CSF 5-HIAA patients scored significantly higher in hostility, but also on several anxiety measures, which is in agreement with Banki's (115) findings, based on anxiety ratings.

There have also been two studies of murderers that suggest that serotonin turnover may be of importance to aggressive acts. Linnoila and co-workers (116) found lower CSF 5-HIAA in impulsive violent offenders than in other types of murderers. Lidberg et al (117) found lower CSF 5-HIAA in those homicide offenders who had killed a spouse or a lover than in those who had killed someone less emotionally cathected (most often a drinking buddy).

The findings in murderers may be relevant for the suicide-serotonin association, since having committed a murder is probably the strongest risk factor of all for ultimate suicide, at least in Western Europe. In Great Britain, a 30% suicide rate is reported after a murder, and it is precisely in those cases where the victim was a spouse that the risk of suicide is greatest (118). (In the United States the suicide rate after murder is lower, around 4%, according to Wolfgang (119).

There is another type of murder which is intimately connected with suicide, and that is the killing of one's own child. Lidberg and co-workers (120) examined three such cases, where a suicide attempter had killed or attempted to kill his or her child. In all three, the CSF 5-HIAA concentrations were very low.

A relationship between serotonin and aggressive behavior was also found by Branchey et al (121), who studied the ratio of tryptophan to other neutral amino acids in serum. They found significantly lower ratios, compatible with a deficiency of brain serotonin, in those subjects who had been arrested for assaultive behavior than in other alcoholics and in nonalcoholic controls.

Serotonin and Alcoholism

Alcoholism in itself may be associated with distrubances in serotonin turnover. Abstinent alcoholics tend to have low concentrations of CSF 5-HIAA (122, 123), and nonalcoholic depressed patients with a family history of alcoholism (depressive spectrum disease according to Winokur (124)) have lower concentrations of CSF 5-HIAA than other depressives (125).

The association with alcohol cannot explain the correlation between low CSF 5-HIAA and suicidal behavior, even if alcohol is often a factor in the suicidal scene. In most studies of suicide attempts and CSF metabolites, alcoholic subjects have been explicitly excluded. It seems more likely that alcohol abuse, and assaultive and suicidal behavior are all part of a syndrome of disinhibitory behavior that might be associated with deficient serotonergic neurotransmission.

Serotonin and Disinhibitory Personality Traits

This hypothesis raises the issue of the possible relationships between serotonin and other, less pathological, aspects of disinhibitory and impulsive behavior. Available evidence (e.g., from personality questionnaire studies) supports a relationship between low CSF 5-HIAA and impulsivity (D Schalling, M Åsberg, G Edman, unpublished data, 1985) and the Validity scale in the Marke-Nyman Temperament Scales (105) and between CSF 5-HIAA and the Psychopathic Deviate scale from the MMPI (59). There are also weak, but consistent correlations with Eysenck's scale Psychoticism, which reflects schizoid, nonconforming, nonempathetic, hostile personality traits (D Schalling, M Åsberg, G Edman, unpublished data, 1985).

IMPLICATIONS FOR SUICIDE PREVENTION

Their association with a heightened risk of suicide suggests that markers of serotonin and HPA activation may be valuable in a clinical context. Low concentrations of CSF 5-HIAA in suicide attempters, for instance, were connected with a 20% mortality from suicide within a year, which suggests that the combination may be one of the strongest suicide predictors hitherto identified.

A dexamethasone test is easy to perform and is unaffected by current antidepressant treatment. In contrast, spinal taps for 5-HIAA measurements require hospitalization and highly standardized procedures, and the patient must not be taking any antidepressant or neuroleptic drugs. There is an obvious need for new, more easily accessible markers of the state of the serotonin system.

A better understanding of the biological and psychological links between serotonin turnover and suicidal behavior might also open up new approaches to the prevention of suicide. Serotonin transmission can be controlled with drugs or amino acid precursors, and possibly by dietary changes, and it would seem important to test such treatment strategies in patients with a high suicide potential. It is also plausible that an increased understanding of the psychological processes that are controlled by serotonin neurons could be used to develop more specific psychotherapeutic techniques than has hitherto been possible.

Acknowledgment. Financial support was given by the Swedish Medical Research Council (5454), The Fredrik and Ingrid Thuring Foundation, The Torsten and Ragnar Söderberg Foundation, The Söderström-König Foundation, and the Karolinska Institute.

The authors would like to thank Richard Pybus and Marie Skjöldebrand for their assistance in the preparation of the manuscript.

References

1. Farberow NL: *Bibliography on Suicide and Suicide Prevention 1897–1957, 1958–1967.* Public Health Service Publication no. 1979. Washington, DC, US Government Printing Office, 1969.
2. Woolley DW, Shaw E: A biochemical and pharmacological suggestion about certain mental disorders. *Proc Natl Acad Sci* 40:228–231, 1954.
3. Schildkraut JJ: The catecholamine hypothesis of affective disorders. A review of supporting evidence. *Am J Psychiatry* 122:509–522, 1965.
4. Lapin IP, Oxenkrug GF: Intensification of the central serotoninergic processes as a possible determinant of the thymoleptic effect. *Lancet* 1:132–136, 1969.
5. Beskow J: Suicide and mental disorder in Swedish men. *Acta Psychiatr Scand*, suppl 277, 1979.
6. Beskow J, Gottfries C-G, Roos B-E, Winblad B: Determination of monoamine and monoamine metabolites in the human brain: post mortem studies in a group of suicides and in a control group. *Acta Psychiatr Scand* 53:7–20, 1976.

7. Carlsson A, Svennerholm L, Winblad B: Seasonal and circadian monoamine variations in human brains examined post mortem. *Acta Psychiatr Scand* 61 (suppl 280):75–83, 1980.

8. Korpi ER, Kleinman JE, Goodman SI, Phillips I, DeLisi LE, Linnoila M, Wyatt RJ: Serotonin and 5-hydroxyindoleacetic acid concentrations in different brain regions of suicide victims: comparison in chronic schizophrenic patients with suicide as cause of death. Presented at the International Society for Neurochemistry, Vancouver, Canada, 1983.

9. Lloyd KG, Farley IJ, Deck JHN, Hornykiewicz O: Serotonin and 5-hydroxyindoleacetic acid in discrete areas of the brainstem of suicide victims and control patients. *Adv Biochem Psychopharmacol* 11:387–397, 1974.

10. Post RM, Ballenger JC, Goodwin FK: Cerebrospinal fluid studies of neurotransmitter function in manic and depressive illness. In Wood JH (ed): *Neurobiology of Cerebrospinal Fluid.* I. New York, Plenum Press, 1980, pp 685–717.

11. Åsberg M, Bertilsson L, Mårtensson B, Scalia-Tomba G-P, Thorén P, Träskman-Bendz L: CSF monoamine metabolites in melancholia. *Acta Psychiatr Scand* 69:201–219, 1984.

12. van Praag HM, Korf J: Endogenous depressions with and without disturbances in the 5-hydroxytryptamine metabolism: a biochemical classification? *Psychopharmacologia* 19:148–152, 1971.

13. Åsberg M, Bertilsson L, Tuck D, Cronholm B, Sjöqvist F: Indoleamine metabolites in the cerebrospinal fluid of depressed patients before and during treatment with nortriptyline. *Clin Pharmacol Ther* 14:277–286, 1973.

14. Åsberg M, Thorén P, Träskman L, Bertilsson L, Ringberger V: "Serotonin depression"—a biochemical subgroup within the affective disorders? *Science* 191:478–480, 1976.

15. Gibbons RD, Davis JM: A note on the distributional form of the Åsberg et al CSF monoamine data. *Acta Psychiatr Scand,* in press, 1985.

16. van Praag HM, de Haan S: Central serotonin metabolism and the frequency of depression. *Psychiatry Res* 1:219–224, 1979.

17. Sedvall G, Fyrö B, Gullberg B, Nybäck H, Wiesel F-A, Wode-Helgodt B: Relationships in healthy volunteers between concentrations of monoamine metabolites in cerebrospinal fluid and family history of psychiatric morbidity. *Br J Psychiatry* 136:366–374, 1980.

18. Sedvall G, Iselius L, Nybäck H, Oreland L, Oxentierna G, Ross SB, Wiesel FA: Genetic studies of CSF monoamine metabolites. Adv Biochem Psychopharmacol 39:79–85, 1984.

19. Wirz-Justice A, Richter R: Seasonality in biochemical determinations: a source of variance and a clue to the temporal incidence of affective illness. *Psychiatry Res* 1:53–60, 1979.

20. Arora RC, Kregel L, Meltzer HY: Seasonal variation of serotonin uptake in normal controls and depressed patients. *Biol Psychiatry* 19:795–804, 1984.

21. Egrise D, Desmedt D, Shoutens A, Mendlewicz J: Circannual variations in the density of tritiated imipramine binding sites on blood platelets in man. *Neuropsychobiology* 10:101–102, 1983.

22. Whitaker PM, Warsh JJ, Stancer HC, Persad E, Vint CK: Seasonal variation in platelet ^{3}H-imipramine binding: comparable values in control and depressed populations. *Psychiatry Res* 11:127–131, 1984.

23. Åsberg M, Bertilsson L, Rydin E, Schalling D, Thorén P, Träskman-Bendz L: Monoamine metabolites in cerebrospinal fluid in relation to depressive illness, suicidal behaviour and personality. In Angrist B, Burrows G, Lader M, Lingjaerde O, Sedvall G, Wheatley D (eds): *Recent Advances in Neuropsychopharmacology.* New York, Pergamon Press, 1981, pp 257–271.

24. Träskman-Bendz L, Åsberg M, Bertilsson L, Thorén P: CSF monoamine metabolites of depressed patients during illness and after recovery. *Acta Psychiatr Scand* 69:333–342, 1984.

25. Schildkraut JJ, Keeler BA, Grab EL, Kantrowich J, Hartmann E: MHPG excretion and clinical classification in depressive disorders. *Lancet* 1:1251–1252, 1973.

26. Beckmann H, Goodwin FK: Urinary MHPG in subgroups of depressed patients and normal controls. *Neuropsychobiology* 6:91–100, 1980.

27. Muscettola G, Potter WZ, Pickar D, Goodwin FK: Urinary 3-methoxy-4-hydroxyphenyl-glycol and major affective disorders—a replication and new findings. *Arch Gen Psychiatry* 41:337–342, 1984.
28. Fernstrom JD, Wurtman RJ: Brain serotonin content: physiological regulation by plasma neutral amino acids. *Science* 178:414–416, 1972.
29. Wood K, Coppen A: Biochemical abnormalities in depressive illness: tryptophan and 5-hydroxytryptamine. In Curzon G (ed): *The Biochemistry of Psychiatric Disturbances.* New York, John Wiley & Sons, 1980, pp 13–33.
30. DeMyer MK, Shea PA, Hendrie HC, Yoshimura NN: Plasma tryptophan and five other amino acids in depressed and normal subjects. *Arch Gen Psychiatry* 38:642–646, 1981.
31. Joseph MS, Brewerton TD, Reus VI, Stebbins GT: Plasma L-tryptophan/neutral amino acid ratio and dexamethasone suppression in depression. *Psychiatry Res* 11:185–192, 1984.
32. Møller SE, Larsen OB: Tryptophan and tyrosine availability: relation to clinical response to antidepressive pharmacotherapy. *Biochem Psychopharmacol* 39:319–326, 1984.
33. Zuckerman M: A biological theory of sensation seeking. In Zuckerman M (ed): *Biological Bases of Sensation Seeking, Impulsivity and Anxiety.* Hillsdale, NJ, Laurence Erlbaum Associates, 1983, pp 37–76.
34. Schalling D, Edman G, Åsberg M: Impulsive cognitive style and inability to tolerate boredom: psychobiological studies of temperamental vulnerability. In Zuckerman M (ed): *Biological Bases of Sensation Seeking, Impulsivity and Anxiety.* Hillsdale, NJ, Lawrence Erlbaum Associates, 1983, pp 123–145.
35. von Knorring L, Oreland L, Winblad B: Personality traits related to monoamine oxidase activity in platelets. *Psychiatry Res* 12:11–26, 1984.
36. Oreland L, Wiberg Å, Åsberg M, Träskman L, Sjöstrand L, Thorén P, Bertilsson L, Tybring G: Platelet MAO activity and monoamine metabolites in cerebrospinal fluid in depressed and suicidal patients and in healthy controls. *Psychiatry Res* 4:21–29, 1981.
37. von Knorring L, Oreland L, Häggendal J, Magnusson T, Almay B, Johansson F: Relationship between platelet MAO activity and concentrations of 5-HIAA and HVA in cerebrospinal fluid in chronic pain patients. *J Neural Transmission,* in press, 1985.
38. Oreland L, Shaskan EG: Monoamine oxidase activity as a biological marker. *Trends Pharmacol Sci* 4:339–341, 1983.
39. Briley MS, Langer SZ, Raisman R, Sechter D, Zarifian E: Tritiated imipramine binding sites are decreased in platelets of untreated depressed patients. *Science* 209:303–305, 1980.
40. Paul SM, Rehavi M, Skolnick P, Ballenger JC, Goodwin FK: Depressed patients have decreased binding of tritiated imipramine to platelet serotonin "transporter." *Arch Gen Psychiatry* 38:1315–1317, 1981.
41. Wägner A, Åberg-Wistedt A, Åsberg M, Montero D, Mårtensson B, Bertilsson L, Ekqvist B: Lower ^{3}H-imipramine binding in platelets from untreated depressed patients compared to controls. *Psychiatry Res,* in press, 1985.
42. Perry EK, Marshall EF, Blessed G, Tomlinson BE, Perry RH: Decreased imipramine binding in the brains of patients with depressive illness. *Br J Psychiatry* 142:188–192, 1983.
43. Tuomisto J, Tukiainen E: Decreased uptake of 5-hydroxytryptamine in blood platelets from depressed patients. *Nature* 262:596–598, 1976.
44. Tuomisto J, Tukiainen E, Ahlfors U-G: Decreased uptake of 5-hydroxytryptamine in blood platelets from patients with endogenous depression. *Psychopharmacology* 65:141–147, 1979.
45. Coppen A, Swade C, Wood K: Platelet 5-hydroxytryptamine accumulation in depressive illness. *Clin Chim Acta* 87:165–168, 1978.
46. Meltzer HY, Arora RC, Baber R, Tricou BJ: Serotonin uptake in blood platelets of psychiatric patients. *Arch Gen Psychiatry* 38:1322–1326, 1981.
47. Malmgren R, Åsberg M, Olsson P, Tornling G, Unge G: Defective serotonin transport mechanism in platelets from endogenously depressed patients. *Life Sci* 29:2649–2658, 1981.
48. Raisman R, Briley MS, Bouchami F, Sechter D, Zarifian E, Langer SZ: ^{3}H-Imipramine binding and serotonin uptake in platelets from depressed patients and control volunteers. *Psychopharmacology* 77:332–335, 1982.

49. Åsberg M, Träskman L, Thorén P: 5-HIAA in the cerebrospinal fluid—a biochemical suicide predictor? *Arch Gen Psychiatry* 33:1193–1197, 1976.
50. Ågren H: Symptom patterns in unipolar and bipolar depression correlating with monoamine metabolites in the cerebrospinal fluid. II. Suicide. *Psychiatry Res* 3:225–236, 1980.
51. Träskman L, Åsberg M, Bertilsson L, Sjöstrand L: Monoamine metabolites in CSF and suicidal behavior. *Arch Gen Psychiatry* 38:631–636, 1981.
52. van Praag HM: Depression, suicide and the metabolism of serotonin in the brain. *J Affective Disord* 4:275–290, 1982.
53. Montgomery SA, Montgomery D: Pharmacological prevention of suicidal behaviour. *J Affective Disord* 4:291–298, 1982.
54. Palanappian V, Ramachandran V, Somasundaram O: Suicidal ideation and biogenic amines in depression. *Indian J Psychiatry* 25:286–292, 1983.
55. Banki CM, Arató M, Papp Z, Kurcz M: Biochemical markers in suicidal patients. Investigations with cerebrospinal fluid amine metabolites and neuroendocrine tests. *J Affective Disord* 6:341–350, 1984.
56. Pérez de los Cobos JZ, López-Ibor Alino JJ, Saiz Ruiz J: Correlatos biológicos del suicidio y la agresividad en depresiones mayores (con melancolía): 5-HIAA en LCR, DST, y respuesta terapéutica a 5-Htp. Presented to the First Congress of the Spanish Society for Biological Psychiatry, Barcelona, 1984.
57. Roy-Byrne P, Post RM, Rubinow DR, Linnoila M, Savard R, Davis D: CSF 5HIAA and personal and family history of suicide in affectively ill patients: a negative study. *Psychiatry Res* 10:263–274, 1983.
58. Ågren H: Life at risk: markers of suicidality in depression. *Psychiatr Dev* 1:87–104, 1983.
59. Brown GL, Ebert MH, Goyer PF, Jimerson DC, Klein WJ, Bunney WE, Goodwin FK: Aggression, suicide, and serotonin: relationships to CSF amine metabolites. *Am J Psychiatry* 139:741–746, 1982.
60. van Praag HM: CSF 5-HIAA and suicide in non-depressed schizophrenics. *Lancet* 2:977–978, 1983.
61. Ninan PT, van Kammen DP, Scheinin M, Linnoila M, Bunney WE Jr, Goodwin FK: CSF 5-hydroxyindoleacetic acid in suicidal schizophrenic patients. *Am J Psychiatry* 141:566–569, 1984.
62. Kauert G, Gilg T, Eisenmenger W, Spann W: Postmortem biogenic amines in CSF of suicides and controls. Presented at the 14th Congress of the Collegium Internationale Neuro-Psychopharmacologicum, Florence, 1984.
63. Garrick NA, Tamarkin L, Taylor PL, Markey SP, Murphy DL: Light and propranolol suppress the nocturnal elevation of serotonin in the cerebrospinal fluid of rhesus monkeys. *Science* 221:474–476, 1983.
64. Stengel E, Cook NC: *Attempted Suicide.* London, Chapman & Hall, 1958.
65. Ettlinger R: Evaluation of suicide prevention after attempted suicide. *Acta Psychiatrica Scand*, suppl 260, 1975.
66. Pokorny AD: Prediction of suicide in psychiatric patients. *Arch Gen Psychiatry* 40:249–257, 1983.
67. Grote SS, Moses SG, Robins E, Hudgens RW, Croninger AB: A study of selected catecholamine metabolizing enzymes: a comparison of depressive suicides and alcoholic suicides with controls. *J Neurochem* 23:791–802, 1974.
68. Mann JJ, Stanley M: Postmortem monoamine oxidase enzyme kinetics in the frontal cortex of suicide victims and controls. *Acta Psychiatr Scand* 69:135–139, 1984.
69. Gottfries C-G, Oreland L, Wiberg Å, Winblad B: Lowered monoamine oxidase activity in brains from alcoholic suicides. *J Neurochem* 25:667–673, 1975.
70. Buchsbaum MS, Coursey RD, Murphy DL: The biochemical high-risk paradigm: behavioral and familial correlates of low platelet monoamine oxidase activity. *Science* 194:339–341, 1976.
71. Buchsbaum MS, Haier RJ, Murphy DL: Suicide attempts, platelet monoamine oxidase and the average evoked response. *Acta Psychiatr Scand* 56:69–79, 1977.
72. Gottfries C-G, von Knorring L, Oreland L: Platelet monoamine oxidase activity in mental

68 / Suicide

disorders. 2. Affective psychoses and suicidal behavior. *Prog Neuro-Psychopharmacol* 4:185–192, 1980.
73. Stanley M, Virgilio J, Gershon S: Tritiated imipramine binding sites are decreased in the frontal cortex of suicides. *Science* 216:1337–1339, 1982.
73a. Paul SM, Rehavi M, Skolnick P, Goowin FK: High affinity binding of antidepressants to a biogenic amine transport site in human brain and platelet: studies in depression. In Post RM, Ballenger JC (eds): *Neurobiology of Mood Disorders.* Baltimore, Williams & Wilkins 1984, pp. 845–953.
74. Meyerson LR, Wennogle LP, Abel MS, Coupet J, Lippa AS, Rauh CE, Beer B: Human brain receptor alterations in suicide victims. *Pharmacol Biochem Behav* 17:159–163, 1982.
75. Stanley M, Mann JJ: Increased serotonin-2 binding sites in frontal cortex of suicide victims. *Lancet* 1:214–216, 1983.
76. Owen F, Cross AJ, Crow TJ, Deakin JFW, Ferrier IN, Lofthouse R, Poulter M: Brain 5-HT₂ receptors and suicide. *Lancet* 2:1256, 1983.
77. Stanley M: Cholinergic receptor binding in the frontal cortex of suicide victims. *Am J Psychiatry* 141:1432–1436, 1984.
78. Kaufmann CA, Gillin JC, Hill B, O'Laughlin T, Phillips I, Kleinman JE, Wyatt RJ: Muscarinic binding in suicides. *Psychiatry* 12:47–55, 1984.
79. Meltzer HY, Umberkoman-Wiita B, Robertson A, Tricou BJ, Lowy M, Perline R: Effect of 5-hydroxytryptophan on serum cortisol levels in major affective disorders. I. Enhanced response in depression and mania. *Arch Gen Psychiatry* 41:366–374, 1984.
80. Meltzer HY, Perline R, Tricou BJ, Lowy M, Robertson A: Effect of 5-hydroxytryptophan on serum cortisol levels in major affective disorders. II. Relation to suicide, psychosis, and depressive symptoms. *Arch Gen Psychiatry* 41:379–387, 1984.
81. Beck-Friis J, Kjellman BF, Aperia B, Undén F, von Rosen D, Ljunggren J-G, Wetterberg L: Serum melatonin in relation to clinical variables in patients with major depressive disorder and a hypothesis of a low melatonin syndrome. *Acta Psychiatr Scand* 71:319–330, 1985.
82. Wetterberg L, Beck-Friis L, Aperia B, Pettersson U: Melatonin/cortisol ratio in depression. *Lancet* 1:1361, 1979.
82a. Claustrat B, Chazot G, Brun J, Jordan D, Sassolas G: A chronobiological study of melatonin and cortisol secretion in depressed subjects: plasma melatonin, a biochemical marker in depression. *Biol Psychiatry* 19:1215–1228, 1984.
83. Banki CM, Vojnik M, Papp Z, Balla KZ, Arato M: Cerebrospinal fluid magnesium and calcium related to amina metabolites, diagnosis and suicide attempts. *Biol Psychiatry* 20:163–171, 1985.
83a. Beckmann H, Wetterberg L, Gattaz WF: Melatonin immunoreactivity in cerebrospinal fluid of schizophrenic patients and healthy controls. *Psychiatry Res* 11:107–110, 1984.
84. Ninan PT, van Kammen DP, Linnoila M: Letter to the editor. *Am J Psychiatry* 142:148, 1985.
85. Ågren H: Biological markers in major depressive disorders. A clinical and multivariate study. Academic dissertation. Acta Universitatis Upsaliensis, Abstracts of Uppsala Dissertations from the Faculty of Medicine 405, Uppsala, 1981.
86. Brown GL, Goodwin FK, Ballenger JC, Goyer PF, Major LF: Aggression in humans correlates with cerebrospinal fluid amine metabolites. *Psychiatry Res* 1:131–139, 1979.
87. Ostroff RB, Giller E, Bonese K, Ebersole E, Harkness L, Mason J: Neuroendocrine risk factors of suicidal behavior. *Am J Psychiatry* 139:1323–1325, 1982.
88. Ostroff RB, Giller E, Harkness L, Mason J: The norepinephrine-to-epinephrine ratio in patients with a history of suicide attempts. *Am J Psychiatry* 142:224–227, 1985.
89. Loosen PT, Prange AJ: Serum thyrotropin response to thyrotropin-releasing hormone in psychiatric patients: a review. *Am J Psychiatry* 139:405–416, 1982.
90. Carroll BJ: The dexamethasone suppression test for melancholia. *Br J Psychiatry* 140:292–304, 1982.
91. Prange AJ Jr, Loosen PT: Peptides in depression. *Adv Biochem Psychopharmacol* 39:127–145, 1984.

92. Bunney WE Jr, Fawcett JA: Possibility of a biochemical test for suicide potential. *Arch Gen Psychiatry* 13:232–239, 1965.
93. Bunney WE Jr, Fawcett JA, Davis JM, Gifford S: Further evaluation of urinary 17-hydroxycorticosteroids in suicidal patients. *Arch Gen Psychiatry* 21:138–150, 1969.
94. Levy B, Hansen E: Failure of the urinary test for suicide potential. Analysis of urinary 17-OHCS steroid findings prior to suicide in two patients. *Arch Gen Psychiatry* 20:415–418, 1969.
95. Krieger G: The plasma level of cortisol as a predictor of suicide. *Dis Nerv Syst* 35:237–240, 1974.
96. Träskman L, Tybring G, Åsberg M, Bertilsson L, Lantto O, Schalling D: Cortisol in the CSF of depressed and suicidal patients. *Arch Gen Psychiatry* 37:761–767, 1980.
97. Brooksbank BWL, Brammall MA, Cunningham AE, Shaw DM, Camps FE: Estimation of corticosteroids in human cerebral cortex after death by suicide, accident or disease. *Psychol Med* 2:56–65, 1972.
98. Carroll BJ, Greden JF, Feinberg M: Suicide, neuroendocrine dysfunction and CSF 5-HIAA concentrations in depression. *Adv Bio-Sci* 31:307–313, 1981.
99. Coryell W, Schlesser MA: Suicide and the dexamethasone suppression test in unipolar depression. *Am J Psychiatry* 138:1120–1121, 1981.
100. Targum SD, Rosen L, Capodanno AE: The dexamethasone suppression test in suicidal patients with unipolar depression. *Am J Psychiatry* 140:877–879, 1983.
101. Robbins DR, Alessi NE: Suicide and the dexamethasone suppression test in adolescence. *Biol Psychiatry* 20:107–110, 1985.
102. Linkowski P, van Wettere JP, Kerkhofs M, Brauman H, Mendlewicz J: Thyrotrophin response to thyreostimulin in affectively ill women: relationship to suicidal behaviour. *Br J Psychiatry* 143:401–405, 1983.
103. Linkowski P, van Wettere JP, Kerkhofs M, Gregoire F, Brauman H, Mendlewicz J: Violent suicidal behavior and the thyrotropin-releasing hormone-thyroid-stimulating hormone test: a clinical outcome study. *Neuropsychobiology* 12:19–22, 1984.
104. Carroll BJ, Greden JF, Haskett R, Feinberg M, Albala AA, Martin FIR, Rubin RT, Heath B, Sharp PT, McLeod WL, McLeod MF: Neurotransmitter studies of neuroendocrine pathology in depression. *Acta Psychiatr Scand* 61 (suppl 280):183–198, 1980.
105. Banki CM, Arató M: Relationship between cerebrospinal fluid amine metabolites, neuroendocrine findings and personality dimensions (Marke-Nyman scale factors) in psychiatric patients. *Acta Psychiatr Scand* 67:272–280, 1983.
105a. Banki CM, Arato M, Papp Z, Kurcz M: The influence of dexamethasone on cerebrospinal fluid monoamine metabolites and cortisol in psychiatric patients. *Pharmacopsychiatria* 16:77–81, 1981.
106. Meltzer HY, Arora RC, Tricou BJ, Fang VS: Serotonin uptake in blood platelets and the dexamethasone suppression test in depressed patients. *Psychiatry Res* 8:41–47, 1983.
107. Gold PW, Goodwin FK, Wehr T, Rebar R: Pituitary thyrotropin response to thyrotropin-releasing hormone in affective illness: relationship to spinal fluid amine metabolites. *Am J Psychiatry* 134:1028–1031, 1977.
108. Bunney WE Jr, Mason JW, Roatch JF, Hamburg DA: A psychoendocrine study of severe psychotic depressive crisis. *Am J Psychiatry* 122:72–80, 1965.
109. Ceulemans DLS, Westenberg HGM, van Praag HM: The effect of stress on the desamethasone suppression test. *Psychiatry Res* 14:189–195, 1985.
110. Anisman H, Pizzino A, Sklar LS: Coping with stress, norepinephrine depletion and escape performance. *Brain Res* 191:583–588, 1980.
111. Valzelli L: *Psychobiology of Aggression and Violence.* New York, Raven Press, 1981.
112. Abraham K: Versuch einer Entwicklungsgeschichte der Libido auf Grund der Psychoanalyse seelischer Störungen. In *Neue Arbeiten zur ärztlichen Psychoanalyse.* Leipzig, Internationaler Psychoanalytischer Verlag, 1927, vol 2.
113. Copenhaver JH, Schalock RL, Carver MJ: *para*-Chloro-D,L-phenylalanine induced filicidal behavior in the female rat. *Pharmacol Biochem Behav* 8:263–270, 1978.
114. Rydin E, Schalling D, Åsberg M: Rorschach ratings in depressed and suicidal patients with

low levels of 5-hydroxyindoleacetic acid in cerebrospinal fluid. *Psychiatry Res* 7:229–243, 1982.

115. Banki CM: Correlation of anxiety and related symptoms with cerebrospinal fluid 5-hydroxyindoleacetic acid in depressed women. *J Neural Transmission* 41:135–143, 1977.

116. Linnoila M, Virkkunen M, Scheinin M, Nuutila A, Rimon R, Goodwin FK: Low cerebrospinal fluid 5-hydroxyindoleacetic acid concentration differentiates impulsive from non-impulsive violent behavior. *Life Sci* 33:2609–2614, 1983.

117. Lidberg L, Tuck JR, Åsberg M, Scalia-Tomba G-P, Bertilsson L: Homicide, suicide and CSF 5-HIAA. *Acta Psychiatr Scand* 71:230–236, 1985.

118. West DJ: *Murder followed by Suicide*. London, Heinemann, 1965.

119. Wolfgang ME: *Patterns in Criminal Homicide*. London, Oxford University Press, 1958.

120. Lidberg L, Åsberg M, Sundqvist-Stensman UB: 5-Hydroxyindoleacetic acid levels in attempted suicides who have killed their children. *Lancet* 2:928, 1984.

121. Branchey L, Branchey M, Shaw S, Lieber C: Depression, suicide and aggression in alcoholics and their relationship to plasma amino acids. *Psychiatry Res* 12:219–226, 1984.

122. Ballenger JC, Goodwin FK, Major LF, Brown GL: Alcohol and central serotonin metabolism in man. *Arch Gen Psychiatry* 36:224–227, 1979.

123. Banki CM: Factors influencing monoamine metabolites and tryptophan in patients with alcohol dependence. *J Neural Transmission* 50:89–101, 1981.

124. Winokur G: The types of affective disorders. *J Nerv Ment Dis* 156:82–96, 1973.

125. Rosenthal NE, Davenport Y, Cowdry RW, Webster MH, Goodwin FK: Monoamine metabolites in cerebrospinal fluid of depressive subgroups. *Psychiatry Res* 2:113–119, 1980.

126. Shaw DN, Camps FE, Eccleston EG: 5-Hydroxytryptamine in the hind-brain of depressive suicides. *Br J Psychiatry* 113:1407–1411, 1967.

127. Bourne HR, Bunney WE Jr, Colburn RW, Davis JM, Davis JN, Shaw DM, Coppen AJ: Noradrenaline, 5-hydroxytryptamine, and 5-hydroxyindoleacetic acid in hindbrains of suicidal patients. *Lancet* 2:805–808, 1968.

128. Pare CMB, Yeung DPH, Price K, Stacey RS: 5-Hydroxytryptamine, noradrenaline and dopamine in brainstem, hypothalamus and caudate nucleus of controls and of patients committing suicide by coal-gas poisoning. *Lancet* 2:133–135, 1969.

129. Cochran E, Robins E, Grote S: Regional serotonin levels in brain: a comparison of depressive suicides and alcoholic suicides with controls. *Biol Psychiatry* 11:283–294, 1976.

130. Åsberg M, Bertilsson L: Serotonin in depressive illness—studies of CSF 5-HIAA. In Saletu B (ed): *Neuropsychopharmacology*. New York, Pergamon Press, 1979, pp 105–115.

131. Wode-Helgodt B, Sedvall G: Correlations between height of subject and concentrations of monoamine metabolites in cerebrospinal fluid from psychotic men and women. *Commun Psychopharmacol* 2:177–183, 1978.

132. Johansson B, Roos B-E: 5-Hydroxyindoleacetic and homovanillic acid levels in the cerebrospinal fluid of healthy volunteers and patients with Parkinson's syndrome. *Life Sci* 6:1449–1454, 1967.

133. Andersen O, Johansson BB, Svennerholm L: Monoamine metabolites in successive samples of spinal fluid—a comparison between healthy volunteers and patients with multiple sclerosis. *Acta Neurol Scand* 63:247–254, 1981.

134. Hallert C, Åström J, Sedvall G: Psychic disturbances in adult coeliac diseases. III. Reduced central monoamine metabolites and signs of depression. *Scand J Gastroenterol* 17:25–28, 1982.

135. Andersson H, Roos B-E: Increased level of 5-hydroxyindoleacetic acid in cerebrospinal fluid from infantile hydrocephalus. *Experientia* 22:539–541, 1966.

136. Bowers MB Jr: Cerebrospinal fluid 5-hydroxyindoleacetic acid (5-HIAA) and homovanillic acid (HVA) following probenecid in unipolar depressives treated with amitriptyline. *Psychopharmacologia* 23:26–33, 1972.

137. Post RM, Goodwin FK: Effects of amitriptyline and imipramine on amine metabolites in the cerebrospinal fluid of depressed patients. *Arch Gen Psychiatry* 30:234–239, 1974.

138. Muscettola G, Goodwin FK, Potter WZ, Claeys MM, Markey SP: Imipramine and desipramine in plasma and spinal fluid. *Arch Gen Psychiatry* 35:621–625, 1978.

139. Träskman L, Åsberg M, Bertilsson L, Cronholm B, Mellström B, Neckers LM, Sjöqvist F, Thorén P, Tybring G: Plasma levels of chlorimipramine and its demethyl metabolite during treatment of depression. Differential biochemical and clinical effects of the two compounds. *Clin Pharmacol Ther* 26:600–610, 1979.

140. Bertilsson L, Tuck JR, Siwers B: Biochemical effects of zimelidine in man. *Eur J Clin Pharmacol* 18:483–487, 1980.

141. Nicoletti F, Raffaele R, Falsaperla A, Paci R: Circadian variation in 5-hydroxyindoleacetic acid levels in human cerebrospinal fluid. *Eur Neurol* 20:834–838, 1981.

142. Losonczy MF, Mohs RC, Davis KL: Seasonal variations of human lumbar CSF neurotransmitter metabolite concentrations. *Psychiatry Res* 12:79–87, 1984.

143. Kaye WH, Ebert MH, Raleigh M, Lake R: Abnormalities in CNS monoamine metabolism in anorexia nervosa. *Arch Gen Psychiatry* 41:350–355, 1984.

144. Post RM, Kotin J, Goodwin FK, Gordon E: Psychomotor activity and cerebrospinal fluid amine metabolites in affective illness. *Am J Psychiatry* 130:67–72, 1973.

145. Nordin C, Siwers B, Bertilsson L: Site of lumbar puncture influences levels of monoamine metabolites. Letter to the editor. *Arch Gen Psychiatry* 39:1445, 1982.

146. Träskman-Bendz L: Depression and suicidal behaviour—a biochemical and pharmacological study. Academic dissertation, Stockholm, 1980.

147. Sjöquist B, Johansson B: A comparison between fluorometric and mass fragmentographic determinations of homovanillic acid and 5-hydroxyindoleacetic acid in human cerebrospinal fluid. *J Neurochem* 31:621–625, 1978.

148. Muskiet FAJ, Jeuring HJ, Korf J Sedvall G, Westerink BHC, Teelken AW, Wolthers BG: Correlations between a fluorimetric and mass fragmentographic method for the determination of 3-methoxy-4-hydroxyphenylacetic acid and two mass fragmentographic methods for the determination of 3-methoxy-4-hydroxyphenylethylene glycol in cerebrospinal fluid. *J Neurochem* 32:191–194, 1979.

149. Major LF, Murphy DL, Lipper S, Gordon E: Effects of clorgyline and pargyline on deaminated metabolites of norepinephrine, dopamine and serotonin in human cerebrospinal fluid. *J Neurochem* 32:229–231, 1979.

150. Coppen A, Prange AJ Jr, Whybrow PC, Noguera R: Abnormalities of indoleamines in affective disorders. *Arch Gen Psychiatry* 26:474–478, 1972.

151. van Praag HM: Significance of biochemical parameters in the diagnosis, treatment, and prevention of depressive disorders. *Biol Psychiatry* 12:101–131, 1977.

152. Leckman JF, Charney DS, Nelson CR, Heninger G, Bowers M: CSF tryptophan, 5-HIAA and HVA in 132 patients characterized by diagnosis and clinical state. *Recent Adv Neuropsychopharmacol* 31:289–297, 1981.

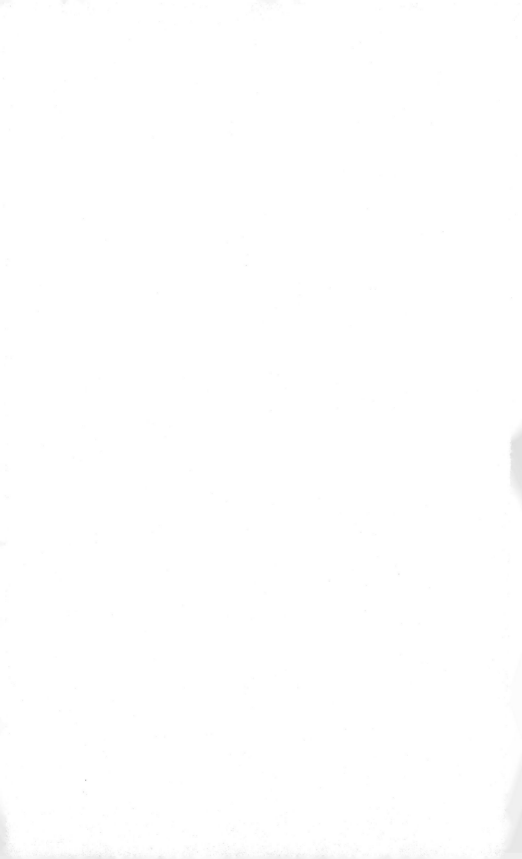

5

Depression, Suicide, and Suicide Prevention

Peter Sainsbury, M.D., F.R.C.P., F.R.C. Psych.

Many writers have been inspired by depression and gloom; and some, such as Robert Burton, positively applauded melancholy, as for instance, when he said "All my joys to this are folly,/ nought so sweet as melancholy." But Burton also recognized its more sinister side, and aptly observed that "black bile is a shoeing-horn to suicide." No textbook of psychiatry conveys the melancholic's feelings as cogently as the mercurial John Donne when he wrote of his emptiness at midnight upon S. Lucies day, being the shortest day " . . . and I am rebegot of absence, darkness, death; things which are not." Other despondent poets have conveyed the unique quality of suicidal despair: Chatterton, who committed suicide, or William Cowper, who tried to and complained "man disavows and Diety disowns me"—a state of mind which psychiatrists more mundanely recognize as "the speech and content of thought of the depressive (I.C.D. 296.1)," and as something that is very different from sadness or unhappiness, however great.

But the association between suicide and depression is something more than a matter of literary interest; it has become one of considerable practical importance. Recent research has not only found that probably the majority of suicides suffered from an unequivocal and treatable depressive illness, but that most of them also contacted their doctors during the period immediately preceding their death. As these observations have urgent implications for suicide prevention, it is proposed to discuss the relations between depresssion and suicide with this preventive aspect in view.

THE INCIDENCE OF SUICIDE IN DEPRESSIVES

The evidence that a high proportion of suicides have a primary depressive illness derives from three sources.

First are studies in which patients with a manic-depressive or endogenous type of depressive illness are followed up. When this is done a consistent finding is that about one in six (15%) of them will die by suicide. Table 5.1 illustrates this. It shows the proportion of deaths from suicide and from other causes in six cohorts followed through a number of years.

More recently, Miles (1) reviewed no less than 30 follow-up studies of patients with a depresive illness, including 7 cohorts of "neurotic depressives." He also reached the conclusion that 15% of depressives, whether classified as endogenous or neurotic, will ultimately die by suicide.

That this figure (of 15%) is probably a valid estimate can be inferred by using it to calculate the expected number of depressed suicides when the life span of a depressive is assumed to be 66 years (2) and the prevalence of severe depression to be about 2% of the population (3). The calculation in Table 5.2 deduces that we can expect about half of England's suicides to be depressives; a proportion that corresponds closely to the figure actually observed in a consecutive sample of clinically assessed suicides (4).

These estimates gain further support from surveys in which the mortality of a population has been recorded over long periods. Helgason (5), for instance, followed a cohort of 5400 Icelanders through 60 or so years. From national records he ascertained that 103, or nearly 2% of the cohort developed a manic-depressive illness; 34 of them died, 18 by suicide. Again, therefore, 17% of the manic-depressives in the cohort comitted suicide. In a more recent prospective study, Hagnell and Rorsman (6) also followed a large cohort of over 3500 residents in Lundby through 15 years. They found that 28 committed suicide, and were able to establish a diagnosis of endogenous depression *in half of them*. They showed that in Sweden, as in England, some 50% of suicides were suffering from a primary depressive illness.

The mortality of manics is relevant too, because most of them enter a depressive phase; and, in fact, when Tsuang and Woolson (7) followed 100 manics through four decades they found that 9% of the decreased had committed suicide, most of them in the first 10 years.

Table 5.1. Death by Suicide in Affective Disorder*

	Cases (No.)	Follow-up (Years)	Dead (No.)	Suicide (No.)	Death Due to Suicide (%)
Langeluddecke (47)	341	40	268	41	15.3
Slater (48)	138	30	59	9	15.3
Lundquist (49)	319	20	119	17	14.3
Schulz (50)	2004	5	492	66	13.4
Stenstedt (51)	216	10	42	6	14.3
Pitts and Winokur (52)	56	Death	56	9	16.0

* Adapted from Robins et al (8).

Table 5.2. Calculation to Obtain Expected Numbers of Depressed Suicides

1. The suicide rate of depressives can be estimated as:

$$\frac{\text{Fraction dying by suicide } (0.15)}{\text{Mean life span of depressives } (66 \text{ years})} \times 10^5 = 230/100,000/\text{year}$$

2. If $2 \pm 0.62\%$ of the 50 million population of England and Wales have a depressive illness, then between 3000 and 1600 suicides with depression can be expected each year, e.g.,

$$\frac{2.62 \times (50 \times 10^6)}{100} \times \frac{230}{10^5} = 3013$$

3. As there are about 5000 suicides/annum, one would then expect between 30 and 60% of them to have a depressive illness.

4. This expected proportion agrees with the 64% of suicides who were observed to have a depression when the 100 suicides in Southern England were clinically assessed.

Depressive Illness in a Sample of Suicides

The second source of evidence for supposing that a high proportion of those who commit suicide already suffered from a primary depressive illness originates from the work of Eli Robins and his team in St. Louis (8). Their method was to undertake diagnostic interviews with the suicides' relatives. From the accounts given by the families of 134 suicides they concluded that 94% had a definite mental disorder and that 45% of them suffered from a manic-depressive illness. Dorpat and Ripley (9), using similar methods, diagnosed 30% of suicides in Seattle as having a depressive disorder.

Barraclough et al (4) embarked on another survey of this kind in West Sussex and Portsmouth. They obtained standardized social as well as clinical data by interviewing the relatives and friends of 100 suicides soon after their deaths, and also 150 controls from the general population. The controls were matched for age, sex, and whether ever married with 75 consecutive suicides. In addition, the suicides' general practitioners provided information on any medical care they had given. The sample was representative insofar as the demographic characteristics of the suicides did not differ from the national figures.

Whether or not each suicide was mentally ill and, if so, what the diagnosis might be were decided by an independent panel of three consultant psychiatrists using these records. The panel agreed that 93% had an identifiable mental disorder and that 64% had an uncomplicated primary depressive illness. This figure increases to 77% if those suicides whose principal diagnosis was alcoholism, but who also had a severe depression, are included (see Table 5.3).

Clinically, most of the 64 depressions were of the endogenous type, but 17% of them had experienced manic episodes as well. Their symptoms were those usually found in depressions of this kind, and they are shown in Table 5.4. But in order to see in what respects the suicidal depressives differed from living ones, they were compared with a random sample of 128 endogenous depressives (matched on age and sex) drawn from the same population as the suicides (10). The rank order of the frequency of 10 leading depressive symptoms was the same for both groups (Table 5.4), though their severity was more often rated higher in the suicides. They differed significantly on only three clinical items: the suicides manifested more persistent insomnia, more self-neglect, and more impairment of memory. Insomnia is important, both because other workers have shown it to be characteristic of the suicidal depressive

Table 5.3. Diagnostic Classification of 100 Suicides

	No. with Principal Diagnosis	No. with Other Diagnosis*
Depressive illness	64	77
Mixed affective state	2	2
Alcoholism*	15	15
Other disorders†	7	7
Schizophrenia	3	3
Diagnosis not possible‡	2	2
Not mentally ill	7	7
Total	100	113

* Ten had alcoholism and depressive illness.
† Two had some other disorder with a depressive illness.
‡ One had depressive illness with another, but undiagnosable condition.

Table 5.4. Clinical Comparisons between Depressed Suicides and Living Depressions (10)

	Suicides (N = 64) (%)	Depressives (N = 128) (%)	χ^2	p
Symptoms:				
Insomnia	84	64	7.57	$p < 0.01$
Self-neglect	17	1	16.90	$p < 0.001$
Impaired memory	17	2	14.12	$p < 0.001$
Depression	95	90	NS*	
Retardation/anergy	47	34	NS	
Loss of concentration	42	45	NS	
Agitated	36	30	NS	
Hypochondriacal	36	29	NS	
Anxious	34	23	NS	
Delusions	9	9	NS	
Other	18	12	NS	
Length of present illness:				
Up to 6 months	55	72		
6 months < 1 year	18	6	16.43	$p < 0.001$
1 year < 2 years	16	4	df = 3	
2 years and more	11	18		
Not known	2	0		
Past history:				
Previous mental illness	44	37	NS	
Previous suicide attempt	41	4	32.28	$p < 0.001$
Family history of mental illness	20	26	NS	

* NS, not significant; df, degrees of freedom.

(11, 12) and because Barraclough et al (13) found that many of the suicides used barbiturates to kill themselves. As the impaired memory and self-neglect were not associated with organic cerebral disease, they probably depict the frequently seen effects of a severe depressive illness on cognitive function and on morale.

Others have compared depressives who committed suicide with diagnostically matched controls; but their suicides were psychiatric admissions and therefore a selected group, and the sources of their data were hospital case notes. McDowall et al (14), for example, assessed the suicides as more severely depressed, but less hypo-chondrical than his controls; and Fareberow and McEvoy (12) rated the suicidal depressives as more agitated. In a more recent study hospital patients diagnosed as having a serious neurotic depression and who had committed suicide were carefully matched on diagnosis with patients who had not (15). Roy then compared the two groups on various items which are systematically recorded in the case notes. He found that significantly more of the suicides were foreign born, unmarried, and living alone. They also not only had more previous admissions than the controls, but were more depressed and suicidal at that time as well. In all of the controlled comparisons, however, the suicides had made *significantly more previous attempts.* Barraclough and Pallis's (10) figures were 41% and 4%; that is, the depressed suicides had made a suicidal attempt 10 times more often than had the living depressives. Another distinctive feature of the depressive who dies by suicide, which has been clearly identified, is that the risk is greater in the period immediately following discharge from hospital (16); a third or more of the suicides occur within 6 months of leaving (17). However, Copas et al (18) found that their deaths are more likely at the start as well as toward the end of an episode of a depressive illness, and when Barraclough et al (4) estimated the duration of their illnesses it was longer in the suicides than in the controls.

Other predisposing factors that distinguished the depressed suicides in Sussex were that they were signficantly more often male, older, separated, socially isolated, and recently bereaved (19); but whereas Bunch et al's (20) sample of suicides did not differ from the general population on early parental bereavement, Roy's (21) hospital suicides did differ from their depressed controls in this respect.

The two groups did *not* differ, however, on number of previous episodes of treated depressive illness—the figure was about 40% in both (see Table 5.4)—nor on family history of mental illness—about 20% of the first-degree relatives of both groups had received treatment for an affective disorder, and 6% of the suicides' relatives had also committed suicide. These figures are not dissimilar to those reported in genetic studies of depressive psychoses. Thus, Perris (22) in his study on the genetics of bipolar or "manic-depressive psychoses" and of unipolar or "recurrent depressive psychoses" reported that the incidence of suicide in the first-degree relatives of bipolar cases was about 16% and in those of unipolar cases it was 11%. These resemblances also tend to confirm the validity of the diagnoses given to the suicides by the panel of psychiatrists. Last, the *social* circumstances of the two depressive groups did not differ as regards unemployment and social class (in both groups the jobless and the wealthier classes were overrepresented as compared with the general population); but they did differ in one very important respect: *42% of the suicides had lived alone*, whereas only 7% of the living depressives did. And this is in keeping with the common epidemiological finding that suicides are generally less well integrated with their neighborhood and domestic group.

The close resemblance between the suicides with depression and a series of depressives with a confirmed diagnosis of endogenous depression again supports the authenticity of the suicides' diagnoses retrospectively determined. The salient inferences, however, are that more than half the suicides have been shown to have a readily identifiable and treatable illness; that their depression has some distinctive clinical features denoting a suicide risk; and, as a corollary of these observations, that there is considerable scope for preventive action.

Depression and Attempted Suicide

A third source of data intimating that suicides are largely recruited from overt depressives, and should therefore be preventable, derives from recent studies on attempted suicide. These have been of two kinds: on the one hand, Bagley (23), Henderson et al (24), and Kiev (25) used the statistical techniques of principal components and cluster analysis to identify categories of attempted suicide. These investigations are consistent in differentiating a psychotically or *severely depressed group* of patients who make a *serious attempt* in circumstances that make discovery unikely. On the other hand, there are studies in which the clinical characteristics of a sample of attempted suicides are related to various measures of the medical seriousness of the attempt or of their *intent to die*. The consensus of 10 such projects is that the clinical variables most positively associated with the seriousness of intent to die are, once more, a diagnosis of manic-depressive or primary depressive illness and a high score on a depression scale. Their conclusions are summarized in Table 5.5. Pallis (26)

Table 5.5. Seriousness of Suicide Attempt in Relation to Clinical and Other Characteristics*

Reference	Year	Variables Associated with Seriousness	
Schmidt et al (53)	1954	Manic depressive, depressive symptoms, dementia	Older age, recent bereavement
Stengel and Cook (54)	1958	Manic depressive, melancholia	
Weiss et al (55)	1961	Depressive or psychotic features	Older age
Dorpat and Boswell (56)	1963	Depression, psychosis	Older age
Rosen (11)	1970	Depression, schizophrenia, organic illness, insomnia	Older, married, widowed, retired, living alone, middle-class and stable residence. Attempt by carbon monoxide, barbiturates, salicylates
Birtchnell and Alarcon (57)	1971	Depressive score; admitted to mental hospital	Male
McHugh and Goodall (58)	1971	Depressive illness	Male
Silver et al (59)	1971	Depressive score	
Minkoff et al (60)	1973	Depressive score	
Pallis and Sainsbury (27)	1976	Depressive symptoms and score	Male, elderly, separated from spouse, living alone

* Adapted from Pallis (26).

inferred that patients making a serious attempt resemble completed suicides rather than attempted suicides in general; and indeed, both he and Rosen (11) have shown that more patients whose attempts are rated as serious subsequently commit suicide than do those whose attempts are rated as less serious.

Pallis (26, 27) for example, clinically assessed 151 consecutive suicide attempts admitted to the emergency department at St. Richard's Hospital in Chichester. Pallis scored each of them on Beck's Intent Scales and on a suicide-risk scale; he also obtained an independent rating of the "medical seriousness" of the attempt from the casualty doctors. Intent to die not only correlated significantly with both suicide risk scores and with medical seriousness ratings, but also with the number and severity of depressive symptoms.

The depressive features that distinguished the high from the low intent suicide attempts are shown in Table 5.6. The two groups also differed significantly on those social variables which have been shown to be strongly associated with consumated suicide, and they are listed in Table 5.7 (27). Once again, the high intent cases were significantly more often males, older, single or separated, and living alone. The depressive and other features of the *serious suicide attempt* are therefore very similar

Table 5.6. Significant Differences between High and Low Intent Groups for Symptoms Experienced in the Last Month (A) and for Behavior at Interview (B)*

Variable	High intent (N = 75)		Low intent (N = 75)		χ^2	p
	No.	%	No.	%		
A. Insomnia	65	87	40	53	18.29	0.01
Pessimism	45	60	24	32	10.73	0.01
Impaired concentration	16	21	3	4	8.68	0.01
Loss of interest	24	32	10	13	6.43	0.02
Social withdrawal	22	29	9	12	5.85	0.02
Feeling useless or worthless	21	28	10	13	4.07	0.05
Weight loss	27	36	15	20	4.00	0.05
B. Slow speech	14	19	3	4	6.63	0.02
Discouraged posture	35	47	19	25	6.22	0.02

* No significant difference between groups:
   A. Depressive mood; worrying; anger/irritability; weeping; anxiety/tension; agitation; appetite; tiredness; self-blame; loss of confidence; depersonalization.
   B. Depressed; anxious/agitated; crying; histrionic; hostile.

Table 5.7. Demographic Characteristics by Level of Intent and Intergroup Differences

	Total Sample (N = 151)	Low (N = 57)	Medium (N = 41)	High (N = 53)
Sex				
Male	35	25	34	47*
Female	65	75	66	53
Age				
15–29	49	54	49	43*
30–44	29	35	27	24
45+	22	10	24	32
Marital status				
Single	34	32	34	38*
Married or cohabiting	41	53	42	28
Divorced-separated-widowed-living apart	24	16	25	33
Living arrangement				
With others	87	96	90	75*
Alone/no fixed abode	12	4	10	25

* The difference between the high and low intent groups was significant (χ^2, $p < 0.05$, 1 df).

to those ascertained by interviewing relatives of *completed* suicides soon after their death.

Pallis and Birtchnell (28) looked at the *seriousness of suicide attempts and personality*. They were able to do this because for a period patients registered on the Northeast of Scotland Psychiatric Case Register routinely completed the Minnesota Multiphasic Personality Inventory (MMPI). They therefore compared the MMPI scores of four samples: 126 nonsuicidal patients, 42 suicide attempts rated serious, 42 attempts rated as not serious, and 14 patients who later died by suicide. Whereas the personality profiles of the suicides and serious attempts were similar and did not differ significantly from the nonsuicidal patients, both differed from the much more deviant profiles of nonserious attempters; the only distinctive feature of the suicides was their high score on introversion.

What has emerged so far is, first, that the seriously suicidal, as well as those who die by suicide, commonly suffer from a primary depression; and second, that attempted suicides in whom the intent to die is rated as serious are not only more likely to have a severe, endogenous type of depression than do those with low intent scores, but they also resemble completed suicides more closely than do attempted suicides in whom intent is low. It is therefore plain that recognizing those patients who have an unequivocal depressive illness is a clinical priority when assessing the likelihood of suicide, and that imparting the skills needed to identify those most at risk must be an essential ingredient of any preventive program.

DEPRESSION AND SUICIDE RISK

Barraclough and Pallis (10) have shown that the clinical similarities between depressed suicides and living depressives are more in evidence than the differences. Accordingly, other factors need to be taken into account in order to specify which patients are most likely to commit suicide.

The evidence not only of these case studies, but also from epidemiological studies is that sociocultural milieu is one important component: both suicides and depressives, for example, tend to have a higher incidence in the more affluent socioeconomic classes and among those who live alone. Another is the *psychosocial stresses and adverse events* to which the individual has recently been exposed—bereavements in the preceding 2 or 3 years have been shown to precipitate both suicide and depression, as have moving house and loss of employment (19, 29–31).

In order to elucidate the interdependence of some of these life stresses, social, and psychological factors, and to pursue the hypothesis that the more closely the individual attempting suicide resembles the completed suicide, the greater the risk of his subsequently killing himself, Pallis et al (32) compared the sample of 75 suicides whose relatives were interviewed with their sample of 146 attempted suicides. They compared them on 55 clinical and social items from the standardized interview schedule that both groups had received. Then, using a stepwise discriminant function analysis, he identified the best discriminators. Two sets of items, one with 18 and the other with 6 variables, enabled 91% and 83% of the combined sample of suicides and attempted suicides to be allocated correctly to their respective groups. That is, the clinical and social information predicted with a high degree of accuracy which of the 221 cases had attempted suicide and which had killed themselves. Once again, it emerged that the items characterizing the completed suicides were those that depicted social isolation and the now familiar clinical and demographic features of the manic-depressive.

On the basis of these findings Pallis constructed a long suicide risk scale (of 18 items) and a shorter one (of 6 items) and then examined their value in screening attempts in the hospital emergency department—that is, as predictors of future suicide in people who had attempted suicide.

To do this 1263 attempted suicides were scored on the sociodemographic and clinical items of the two risk scales (weighted according to their value in discriminating between suicides and attempted suicides). The attempted suicides were also rated on an "intent to die" scale. All of the cases were then followed up for 2 years. Ten of the 12 suicides occurring in the first year were patients who were in the top quartile of the 6-item scale. The 18-item one was even more efficient, but the predictive efficiency was further improved by also taking into account the ratings of intent to die (33). The practical implications of these studies are that intent and risk scales not only point to the severely depressed, whether categorized as endogenous or neurotic, as being highly vulnerable, but that they can also efficiently predict the short term risk of suicide. Hence they have potential value in quickly assessing the management of suicide attempts, and so in the *prevention* of suicide. Indeed, the feasibility of prevention largely depends on the ability of the primary care services: (*a*) to recognize the depressed patient and those of his characteristics which denote a suicide risk; (*b*) to provide effective antidepressant treatment; and (*c*) to organize efficient aftercare. A number of evaluative studies were undertaken to see how effectively the suicidally depressed are identified and managed by services; and they can be quoted to support these three contentions.

PRIMARY CARE OF DEPRESSIVE SUICIDES

This discussion will begin by considering the warnings and threats that Barraclough et al's (4) 100 suicides gave of their intentions: 53% of the 64 uncomplicated depressives made an unequivocal threat of suicide in the month before death, and nearly half of the alcoholic depressives also did.

But of greater preventive relevance was their further observation that over 60% of the depressives contacted their general practitioner in the month before their death (see Table 5.8). And, surprisingly, a high proportion of depressed *suicide attempters* are also reported (26, 34) to have seen their doctors just prior to the act. It is apparent that with the majority of suicidal depressives there are ample opportunities for intervention, providing the doctor has the required skills to take advantage of them. It is of interest, therefore, to see how the Sussex general practitioners in 1966 managed the suicidal depressives, and hence whether prevention is a practicable proposition.

Eighty-one percent of the suicides had been prescribed hypnotics and tranquilizers (see Table 5.9), so in the large majority their doctors recognized that they were distressed. But only 30% had been given antidepressants and in only 1 of the 19 given antidepressants were the dosage and type appropriate. Furthermore, over half had been prescribed barbiturates, and half of the depressives dying from barbiturates had received the tablets in the previous week, all but two using the prescribed tablets to commit suicide (13).

Clearly, in 1966, when the suicides' general practitioners and families were visited, there was a need for more expertise in the primary care of suicidal depressives; but there are grounds for saying that their recognition and management may have changed with the greater emphasis postgraduate education now gives to psychiatry.

Table 5.8. Period between Most Recent Medical Contact and Death for 64 Suicides Diagnosed as Depressive

	Family Doctor (%)	Psychiatrist* (%)	Most Recent Contact of Either (%)
0–7 days	34	9	42
8–30 days	19	8	20
31–90 days	16	3	17
91–365 days	13	2	11
366+ days	17		9
Total	99	22	99

* Total under psychiatric care = 22
  Not under psychiatric care = 78.

Table 5.9. Prescribed Medical Treatment at Time of Death for 64 Suicides Diagnosed as Depressive

Treatment	%
Prescribed psychotropic drugs	81
Barbiturates	53
Antidepressants	30
Phenothiazines	20
Minor tranquilizers	23
Electroconvulsive therapy	5
Haloperiodol	2
Hypnotics	70

While seeking explanations for the recent decline in suicide in England, one of the possibilities Sainsbury et 1 (35) considered was that it could be ascribed to improved mental health services, especially to better primary care by general practitioners. Jenkins (36) therefore compared the consultation rates and diagnoses recorded in two large scale surveys of general practice in England; one was done in *1955 to 1956* and the other in *1970 to 1971* (37, 38).

He found that whereas the consultation rates for *all* conditions fell in the later period, those for psychiatric disorder increased by 60%. Second, the general practitioners' diagnoses in the more recent period were more in accordance with psychiatric conventions. Third, the number of patients being recognized as suffering from disorders with a high suicide risk had greatly increased, especially depressive disorders, as can be seen in Table 5.10. He tentatively inferred that general practitioners' recognition of and attitude toward the depressive patient are probably changing in a direction that could curtail suicide.

THE MANAGEMENT OF THE SUICIDAL DEPRESSIVE BY PSYCHIATRIC SERVICES

Next, the practicability of applying advances in the treatment of depression to suicide prevention can be well illustrated by considering the potential benefits of lithium clinics. Lithium carbonate, it is maintained, prevents relapses in recurrent depression. Using the criteria of recurrence and the success rate that Coppen et al (39) reported in a controlled trial of the prophylactic value of lithium in recurrent depression, Barraclough (40) identified 21 recurrent depressives in his sample of suicides who would have qualified for that trial. He then calculated that had these depressives been treated with lithium as successfully as had the trial patients, a fifth of the suicides would have been prevented; extrapolating to the country as a whole, there would have been 750 fewer suicides.

The management of depressives by psychiatrists is equally in need of reappraisal: too many depressives in psychiatric treatment commit suicide. As Greenblatt (41) and others (42) have shown, the quickest and surest way of removing the suicidal depressive from danger is still by admission to hospital, and often by giving electroconvulsive therapy; despite this a number of studies report that suicides not only received less electroconvulsive therapy than other depressives and spent less time in hospital, but that they also antagonized the staff more (12, 43, 44).

These problems of management of the suicidal patient led Pallis (26) to question general practitioners, psychiatrists, nurses, and Samaritans, both about their attitudes toward the suicidal patient and their knowledge of factors that affect the risk of suicide.

Table 5.10. General Practice Morbidity Study*

A. General Practice Consulting Rates

	1956	1971	% Change
Consulting Rate per 1000			
All diseases or conditions	3751.0	3009.6	−19.8
Mental disorder	187.4	297.6	+58.8
Patient Consulting Rate per 1000			
All diseases or conditions	670	671.1	+1
Mental disorders	50	109.9	+119.8

B. Patient Consulting Rates (per 1000) for Various Selected Diagnoses All Ages, Total Male and Female

	ICD No.	1956	1971	% Change
Anxiety neurosis	300.0	23.1	34.0	+47.2
Depressive neurosis	300.4	1.4	31.4	+2142.9
Neurasthenia	300.5	5.7	2.3	−59.6
Other and unspecified	300.6–300.9	7.0	0.7	−90

* Data from Office of Population Censuses and Surveys (37) and Logan and Cushion (38).

Only the psychiatrists considered that the responsibility for preventing suicide lay with them; and though most respondents believed a depressive illness increases the risk of suicide, they were unaware of most other risk factors. Further, Barraclough found very few of the suicidally depressed contact social and lay services, so that the task of prevention remains largely with family doctors and psychiatrists.

The suicide rates of *resident* psychiatric patients in England (35) have shown a disturbing increase, and one which coincides with the introduction of more liberal regimes in hospitals; de Graaf (45) has reported a similar finding in Holland. Whether the present preference for early discharge and for treating depressives in the community places the suicidal patient at greater risk has yet to be decided. In any case, we now have sufficient facts to formulate realistic plans for the preventive management of the suicidal inpatient. We know that the danger of suicide relates to the onset of a depression and to its duration, and that it also increases in the weeks following discharge from active treatment (15): the importance of supervision while in hospital and of subsequent support in the community are therefore evident.

Walk (46) has given evidence that a well organized community psychiatric service might, in fact, be able to reduce the suicide rate. He compared the suicide rates of all patients in contact with a psychiatrist during the 5 years before and after the introduction of the Chichester Community Psychiatric Service in which 86% of all referrals were treated extramurally. He found a significant decrease in the suicide rate of elderly psychiatric *patients.* Since it was the aged, depressed patients who had benefited most and whose level of referral had increased most after starting community care, there is a likelihood that the new services were responsible.

Management and Prevention

How then, in summary, can doctors, nurses, psychologists, and other service personnel contribute to the prevention of suicide? And how might services be organized to meet this end? Sufficient attention has already been drawn to the first requirement; namely, that doctors, and that usually means the family doctor, should be able to recognize not just those conditions which carry a high risk of suicide, but also the clinical and social characteristics that predispose to the act: these are listed in Table 5.11. This entails being adept at diagnosing depression and the guises it adopts: the smiling depressive, for example, or the patient atypically preoccupied with some bodily symptom, or the unduly taciturn and surly individual, and so forth.

A further prerequisite is to become practiced in broaching the patient's feeling about ending his life, about death and the future. The patient who is in earnest will be relieved by having an opportunity to express his fears. Another crucial part of the assessment of anyone who has made a suicidal attempt is to gauge whether the

Table 5.11. Assessment of the Suicidal: Some Factors Affecting the Risk

1. Personal and social
   M > F: aged over 40;
   Marital status: widowed, divorced, or separated;
   Immigrant;
   Mode of living: alone, does not belong to a domestic group;
   Occupation: unoccupied or unemployed, works in recreational services, retired;
   District: socially disorganized urban areas, resort towns.
2. Previous history
   Family history of affective disorder, suicide, alcoholism;
   Previous history of affective disorder, alcoholism;
   Previous suicide attempt;
   Soon after onset: at the beginning of treatment, 6/12 following discharge from
       active treatment.
3. Life stresses
   Bereavement and separations, moving house, loss of job;
   In alcoholics, domestic and social complications of drinking;
   Incapacitating terminal illness in elderly.
4. Personality
   Cyclothymic, sociopathic (impulsive, violent, capricious, delinquent);
   Excessive drinking and drug dependency.
5. Psychiatric illness
   Depression, notably manic-depressive and recurrent depression;
   Alcoholism and other addictions;
   Early dementia and confusional states in elderly;
   Organic brain syndromes (epilepsy and head injury);
   Combinations of the above.
6. Symptoms
   Depressive: persistent insomnia; dejected appearance and loss of weight, slowed
       speech;
   Loss of usual interests, listlessness and social withdrawal;
   Hopelessness and pessimism;
   Ideas of unworthiness;
   Agitation and restlessness;
   Suicidal thoughts;
   Alcoholics: medical and CNS complications.
7. Circumstances of an attempt
   Precautions taken against discovery;
   Preparatory acts: procuring means, affairs in order, warning statements, suicide
       note;
   Violent methods and more lethal drugs/poisons.

intention to die was serious; and an evaluation of the circumstances in which the attempt was made may provide objective clues to this (see Table 5.11).

Last, effective prevention depends not only on the efficient pharmacological and psychological treatment of the depressive patient, but also on devising a systematic policy for his aftercare; this, of course, also goes for the depressed alcoholic and other high risk patients. If suicide prevention is to become a practicable reality, therefore, the medical and social services need to be organized so as to attain this goal.

In Britain the general practitioner is seen, both by the suicidally disposed and by the relatives, as the person to turn to for help, so it is around him or his equivalent elsewhere that services should pivot. First, he must have effective channels for taking action. This entails having privileged access to the emergency services, such as ambulances and the poisoning treatment center, as well as reliable links with psychiatric and psychological services so that he can quickly obtain a clinical assessment or arrange admission when he needs to. The psychiatric amenities must similarly be available to the emergency treatment center to advise on attempted suicides who are referred there directly, and to provide inpatient care or specialized treatment, such as electroconvulsive therapy, for the severely depressed.

It is for these depressed patients especially that prevention is a goal which a psychiatric multidisciplinary team should be able to realize. Such a team might include psychiatrist, social worker, psychologist, and community nurse, and they would also need to collaborate with the primary care services, such as the general practitioner. The team would then need to evolve a dependable scheme for assessing and supervising the suicide-prone patient during his stay in hospital and particularly during follow-up in the community after discharge.

The responsibility for supporting the patient in the community can be allocated to any member of the team who has a good relationship with the patient and who has the appropriate skills. Thus the care of an uncomplicated depressive on antidepressants, who needs regular monitoring and reassurance following discharge, might fall to the general practitioner; in this context, collaboration with the patient's family can also be valuable. The relapsed depressive is disinclined to seek help; but the relatives can be taught to recognize the clinical features of a relapse and are encouraged to refer the patient back to his doctor if the signs recur. The psychiatrist, on the other hand, might take on the recurrent depressive who needs prophylactic lithium, and he or the psychologist might be allocated patients for whom psychotherapy is indicated, such as the depressed suicide attempter with a neurotic component. The social worker can most aptly deal with the domestic crises that so often precipitate depressive episodes and acts of self-poisoning. The salient requisite, however, is that the patient definitely knows to whom he can turn and depend on for support.

In conclusion, the available facts on the relation of suicide to depression, on the characteristics of the suicidal depressive, and on the opportunities we have for providing effective treatment are such that a substantial proportion of suicides can reasonably be considered as preventable. We should now accept that it should be mandatory to organize preventive policies for the affectively disordered by developing services to provide systematic support for them, and should recognize our responsibility to protect depressives at those times when they are most vulnerable.

References

1. Miles CP: Conditions predisposing to suicide: a review. *J Nerv Ment Dis* 16:231–246, 1977.
2. Oltman JE, Friedman S: Life cycles in patients with manic-depressive psychosis. *Am J Psychiatry* 119:174–177, 1962.

86 / *Suicide*

3. Wing JK: A technique for studying psychiatric morbidity in in-patient and out-patient series and in general population samples. *Psychol Med* 6:665–671, 1976.
4. Barraclough B, Bunch J, Nelson B, Sainsbury P: A hundred cases of suicide: clinical aspects. *Br J Psychiatry* 125:355–373, 1974.
5. Helgason T: The epidemiology of mental disorder in Iceland. *Acta Psychiatr Scand* 40(suppl 173), 1964.
6. Hagnell O, Rorsman B: Suicide and endogenous depression with somatic symptoms in the Lundby study. *Neuropsychobiology* 4:180–187, 1978.
7. Tsuang MT, Woolson RF: Excess mortality in schizophrenia and affective disorders. *Arch Gen Psychiatry* 35:1181–1185, 1978.
8. Robins E, Murphy GE, Wilkinson RH, Gassner S, Kayes J: Some clinical considerations in the prevention of suicide based on a study of 134 sucessful suicides. *Am J Public Health* 49:888–898, 1959.
9. Dorpat T, Ripley HS: A study of suicide in the Seattle area. *Compr Psychiatry* 1:349–359, 1960.
10. Barraclough BM, Pallis D: Depression followed by suicide: a comparison of depressed suicides with living depressives. *Psychol Med* 5:55–61, 1975.
11. Rosen DH: The serious suicide attempt: epidemiological and folllow-up study of 886 patients. *Am J Psychiatry* 127:764–770, 1970.
12. Farberow NL, McEvoy TC: Suicide among patients with diagnosis of anxiety reaction or depressive reaction in general medicinal and surgical hospitals. *J Abnorm Psychol* 71:287–299, 1966.
13. Barraclough B, Nelson B, Bunch J, Sainsbury P: Suicide and barbiturates prescribing. *J R Coll Gen Pract* 21:645–653 1971.
14. McDowall AWT, Brooke EM, Freeman-Browne DL, Robin AA: Subsequent suicide in depressed in-patients. *Br J Psychiatry* 114:749–754, 1968.
15. Roy A: Suicide in depressives. *Comp Psychiatry* 24:487–491, 1983.
16. Pokorny, AD: Suicide rates in various psychiatric disorders. *J Nerv Ment Dis* 139:499–506, 1964.
17. Temoche A, Pugh T, MacMahon B: Suicide rates among current and former mental institution patients. *J Nerv Ment Dis* 138:124–130, 1964.
18. Copas JB, Freeman-Browne DL, Robin AA: Danger periods for suicide in patients under treatment. *Psychol Med* 1:400–44, 1971.
19. Bunch J, Barraclough B, Nelson B, Sainsbury P: Suicide following bereavement of parents. *Soc Psychiatry* 6:193–199, 1971.
20. Bunch JS, Barraclough BM, Nelson B, Sainsbury P: Early parental bereavement and suicide. *Soc Psychiatry* 4:200–202, 1971.
21. Roy A: Suicide in recurrent affective disorder patients. *Can J Psychiatry* 29:319–322, 1984.
22. Perris C: A study of bi-polar (manic depressive) and unipolar recurrent depressive psychoses. *Acta Psychiatr Scand* 42(suppl 194), 1966.
23. Bagley C: Social policy and the prevention of suicidal behaviour. *Br J Soc Work* 3:473–495, 1973.
24. Henderson AS, Hartigan J, Davidson J, Lance GN, Duncan-Jones P, Koller KM, Ritchie K, McAuley H, Williams CL, Slaghuis W: A typology of parasuicide. *Br J Psychiatry* 131:631–641, 1977.
25. Kiev A: Cluster analysis profiles of suicide attempters. *Am J Psychiatry* 133:150–153, 1976.
26. Pallis DJ: The psychiatric assessment of attempted suicide: personality, intent and suicide risk. Thesis, University of Aberdeen, 1977.
27. Pallis DJ, Sainsbury P: The value of assessing intent in attempted suicide. *Psychol Med* 6:487–492, 1976.
28. Pallis DJ, Birtchnell J: Seriousness of suicide attempt in relation to personality. *Br J Psychiatry* 130:253–259, 1977.
29. Sainsbury P, Collins J: Some factors relating to mental illness in a New Town. *J Psychosom Res* 10:45–51, 1966.
30. Sainsbury P: Suicide: opinions and facts. *Proc R Soc Med* 66:579–587, 1973.

31. Paykel ES: Life stress and psychiatric disorder: applications of the clinical approach. In Dohrenwend BS, Dohrenwend BP (eds): *Stressful Life Events: Trait Nature and Effects.* New York, John Wiley & Sons, 1974.
32. Pallis DJ, Barraclough BM, Levey AB, Jenkins J, Sainsbury P: Estimating suicide risk among attempted suicides. I. Development of new clinical scales. *Br J Psychiatry* 141:37–44, 1982.
33. Pallis DJ, Gibbons JS, Pierce DW: Estimating suicide risk among attempted suicides. II. Efficiency of predictive scales after the attempt. *Br J Psychiatry* 144:139–148,1984.
34. Bancroft J, Skrimshire A, Casson J, Harvard-Watts O, Reynolds F: People who deliberately poison or injure themselves: their problems and their contacts with helping agencies. *Psychol Med* 7:289–303, 1977.
35. Sainsbury P, Baert A, Jenkins J: Suicide trends in Europe: a study of the decline in suicide in England and Wales and of the increase elsewhere. A Report to the World Health Organization Regional Office for Europe, Copenhagen, 1978.
36. Jenkins JS: An ecological examination of the social relations of the suicide rates of 18 European countries 1961–63 to 1972–76. Doctoral thesis, Sussex University, 1984.
37. Office of Population Censuses and Surveys: Studies on medical and population subjects. Morbidity Statistic from General Practice. Second National Study 1970–71. London, Her Majesty's Stationery Office, 1974.
38. Logan WPD, Cushion AA: Studies on medical and population subjects. Morbidity Statistics from General Practice. London, General Register Office. Her Majesty's Stationery Office, 1958.
39. Coppen A, Noguera R, Bailey J, Burns BH, Swami MS, Hare EH, Gardener R, Maggs R: Prophylactic lithium in affective disorders. *Lancet* 2:275–279, 1971.
40. Barraclough B: Suicide prevention, recurrent affective disorder and lithium. *Br J Psychiatry* 121:391–392, 1972.
41. Greenblatt M: Efficacy of ECT in affective and schizophrenic illness. *Am J Psychiatry* 13:1001–1005, 1977.
42. Medical Research Council: Report by Clinical Psychiatry Committee. Clinical trial of the treatment of depressive illness. *Br Med J* 1:881–886, 1965.
43. Flood RA, Seager CP: A retrospective examination of psychiatric case records of patients who subsequently committed suicide. *Br J Psychiatry,* 114:443–450, 1968.
44. Robin AA, Brooke EM, Freeman-Browne DL: Some aspects of suicide in psychiatric patients in Southend. *Br J Psychiatry* 114:739–747, 1968.
45. de Graaf AC: Zelfmoord in Psychiatrische Zeikenhuizen. *Tijdsch Psychiatrie* 18:11–12, 1976.
46. Walk D: Suicide and community care. *Br J Psychiatry* 113:1381–1391, 1967.
47. Langeluddecke A: Uber Lebenserwartung und Rucksfallhaufigkeit bei Manisch-depressiven. *Psychiatr Hyg* 13:1–14, 1941.
48. Slater E: Zur Erbpathologie des manish-de-pressiven Irreseins: Die Eltern and Kindern von Manisch Depressiven. *Z Gesamte Neurol Psychiatr* 163:1–47, 1938.
49. Lundquist G: Prognosis and course in manic-depressive psychoses. *Acta Psychiatr Neurol Scand Suppl* 35:1–96, 1945.
50. Schulz B: Sterblichkeit endogen Geisteskranker und Ihrer Eltern. *Z Menschl Vererb Konstitutions Lehre* 29:338–367, 1949.
51. Stenstedt A: A study in manic-depresive psychosis, clinical, social and genetic investigations. *Acta Psychiatr Neurol Scand Suppl* 79:1–111, 1952.
52. Pitts FN, Winokur G: Affective disorder. III. Diagnostic correlates and incidence of suicide. *J Nerv Ment Dis* 139:176–181, 1964.
53. Schmidt EH, O'Neal P, Robins E: Evaluation of suicide attempts as a guide to therapy: clinical and follow-up study of 109 patients. *JAMA* 155:549–557, 1954.
54. Stengel E, Cook N: *Attempted Suicide: Its Social Significance and Effects.* Maudsley Monograph no. 4. London, Chapman and Hall, 1958.
55. Weiss, JMA, Nunez N, Schaie KW: Quantification of certain trends in attempted suicide. In Proceedings of the Third World Congress of Psychiatry, Montreal 1961, pp 1236–1240.
56. Dorpat TL, Boswell JW: An evaluation of suicide intent in suicide attempts. *Compr*

Psychiatry 4:117–125, 1963.

57. Birtchnell J, Alarcon J: Depression and attempted suicide: a study of 91 cases seen in a casualty department. *Br J Psychiatry* 118:289–296, 1971.

58. McHugh PR, Goodell H: Suicidal behaviour: a distinction of patients with sedative poisoning seen in a general hospital. *Arch Gen Psychiatry* 25:456–464, 1971.

59. Silver MA, Bohnert M, Beck AT, Marcus D: Relation of depression to attempted suicide and seriousness of intent. *Arch Gen Psychiatry* 25:573–576, 1971.

60. Minkoff K, Bergman E, Beck AT: Hopelessness, depression and attempted suicide. *Am J Psychiatry 130:455–459, 1973.*

6

Suicide in Alcoholism

George E. Murphy, M.D.

"Get out! I told you when I let you come back that if you ever got drunk and tried to abuse me again, we were through. I meant it. Now, pack your bags and go. I never want to see you again!" The man started to pack, still drinking. Then he shot and killed himself.

Alcoholism, by its nature, leads to strife. Some alcoholics drink all day every day. Some drink only after work. Others drink the weekend away. Others have periods of heavy drinking interspersed with periods of abstinence. Some alcoholics are happy while drinking and morose at other times. Some, pleasant when sober, become self-pitying or belligerent when they drink. Others become expansive, garrulous, or abusive. Abuse is usually restricted to a spouse or paramour, but may include children, employees, or strangers. Whatever the pattern, conflict is a part of it—conflict with a spouse or lover, with the family, with friends, with an employer or foreman, with the police, with drinking companions or with strangers. Frequently there are health problems and economic problems as well.

The *Diagnostic and Statistical Manual of Mental Disorders*, third edition (DSM-III) (1), distinguishes alcohol abuse from alcohol dependence. The practical or clinical reasons for this distinction are unclear. The diagnostic criteria for alcohol abuse require evidence both of a pattern of pathological alcohol use and impairment of occupational functioning due to alcohol use, as well as a minimum duration of 1 month. Criterion symptoms are as follows:

Alcohol Abuse (1, pp 169–170)

A. Pattern of pathological alcohol use
1. Need for daily use of alcohol for adequate functioning
2. Inability to cut down or stop drinking
3. Repeated efforts to control drinking by "going on wagon" or restricting drinking to certain times of the day
4. Binges
5. Occasional consumption of a fifth of spirits (or its equivalent in wine or beer)
6. Amnesic periods for events occurring while intoxicated (blackouts)
7. Drinking nonbeverage alcohol
B. Impairment of social or occupational function due to alcohol use
1. Violence while intoxicated
2. Absence from work
3. Loss of a job
4. Legal difficulties (arrests for intoxicated behavior, traffic accidents while intoxicated)

5. Arguments or difficulties with family or friends because of excessive alcohol use

C. Duration of disturbance of at least 1 month

The diagnostic criteria for *alcohol dependence* require evidence of *either* a pathological pattern of use of alcohol *or* impairment of social or occupational functioning, plus evidence of either tolerance to alcohol or withdrawal symptoms.

Alcohol Dependence (1, p 170)

A. Either a pattern of alcohol use or impairment in social or occupational functioning due to alcohol use:

Pattern of pathological alcohol use:

1. Need for daily use of alcohol for adequate functioning
2. Inability to cut down or stop drinking
3. Repeated efforts to control drinking by "going on wagon" or restricting drinking to certain times of the day
4. Binges
5. Occasional consumption of a fifth of spirits (or its equivalent in wine or beer)
6. Amnesic periods for events occurring while intoxicated (blackouts)
7. Drinking nonbeverage alcohol

Impairment of social or occupational functioning due to alcohol use:

1. Violence while intoxicated
2. Absence from work
3. Loss of a job
4. Legal difficulties (arrests for intoxicated behavior, traffic accidents while intoxicated)
5. Arguments or difficulties with family or friends because of excessive alcohol use.

B. Either tolerance or withdrawal

Tolerance: Need for markedly increased amounts of alcohol to achieve the desired effect, or markedly diminished effect with regular use of the same amount.

Withdrawal: Development of alcohol withdrawal (e.g., morning "shakes" and malaise relieved by drinking) after cessation of or reduction in drinking.

Duration of the problem is not specified, but is perhaps implicit in the tolerance-withdrawal criterion. It is of interest that no minimum number of symptoms is specified in either definition.

This author used a rather more restrictive set of criteria for a diagnosis of alcoholism: those of the Department of Psychiatry of the Washington University School of Medicine. These criteria are listed below. They require at least one symptom in three of the four categories: physical consequences, control problems, legal/vocational trouble, and personal/interpersonal distress.

Alcoholism (2)

For a "definite" diagnosis," symptoms must occur in at least three of the four following groups. A "probable" diagnosis is made when symptoms occur in only two groups.

A. Group One:

1. Any manifestastion of alcohol withdrawal such as tremulousness, convulsions, hallucinations, or delirium
2. History of medical complications, e.g., cirrhosis, gastritis, pancreatitis, myopathy, polyneuropathy, Wernicke-Korsakoff syndrome

3. Alcoholic blackouts
4. Alcoholic binges or benders (48 hours or more of drinking associated with default of usual obligations, occurring more than once)

B. Group Two:
   1. Patient unable to stop drinking when he wanted to
   2. Patient has tried to control drinking by allowing himself to drink only under certain circumstances, such as only after 5:00 p.m., only on weekends, or only with other people
   3. Drinking nonbeverage forms of alcohol

C. Group Three:
   1. Arrests for drinking
   2. Traffic difficulties associated with drinking
   3. Trouble at work because of drinking
   4. Fighting associated with drinking

D. Group Four:
   1. Patient thinks he drinks too much
   2. Family objects to his drinking
   3. Loss of friends because of drinking
   4. Other people object to his drinking
   5. Feels guilty about his drinking

Alcoholism contributes about 25% of the total of suicides in the United States (3, 4). Depending on the population studied, this proportion has been found to be only a little higher or lower in other studies abroad (5–7). In any event, the contribution is a substantial one and second only to that made by depressive illness. Typically, suicide is not an early outcome of alcoholism. In one large study, the mean duration of excessive drinking was 20 years (3). There are relatively few alcoholic suicides in their twenties and thirties, and again few beyond the age of 60. Women comprise only about one-sixth of the total. In this, as in suicides overall, their rate is less than half that of males.

Alcoholics frequently threaten suicide. A rather large number make suicide attempts. Among a series of 50 alcoholic suicides Murphy et al studied, 30% were reported to have done so (8). In this same series, 92% were found to have had a history of communication of suicidal thinking. More than half had first talked it over a year before their death. In some, it had occurred off and on for many years, while in only 12% was communication of this type entirely limited to the final 6 weeks of life. Although critical data are lacking, it appears that suicidal thoughts and communication (including suicide attempts) are frequent among alcoholics in general. For that reason, the significance of any particular communication is difficult to assess unless there is a crisis. Even then, a substantial preoccupation with suicide may not lead to the act. Just what does is a matter of some interest.

Of a consecutive series of 134 urban suicides, 31 of them met criteria for alcoholism (3). Apart from the chronic drinking, one striking feature of this group was a surprisingly high frequency of interpersonal conflict and disruption of interpersonal relationships (9). Half had experienced loss of a close interpersonal relationship within a year before their death. In contrast, this occurred in fewer than 20% of those with a depressive illness who took their lives.

More striking than the year-long accumulation of such circumstances, one of three alcoholics had experienced the disruption of a close interpersonal relationship *within 6 weeks or less* of their self-inflicted death. If there were no relationship between these disruptions and suicide, one would expect them to be evenly distributed among the eight and two-thirds 6-week periods in the year. Instead, there was a highly significant ($p < 0.01$) concentration of such events in the final 6 weeks. Could there be an etiologic relationship between loss of a close personal relationship and suicide among the alcoholics? It did not seem to hold for those with major depression uncomplicated by alcoholism.

Because this was a chance finding, it was uncertain whether it represented a true association. To test that possibility Murphy et al studied an additional 50 alcoholic suicides in the same way (8). In order to avoid biasing the outcome, they were careful to ask no leading questions. As in the original study, informants were systematically asked whether any of a list of potentially stressful events had occurred within a year prior to the death of the victim. For any item answered affirmatively, a date of occurrence was requested. This was recorded, and later calculated against the known date of death. Again, half of the alcoholics had experienced a major interpersonal loss within a year of their death. Those interpersonal disruptions were once again found to be concentrated in the final 6 weeks of their lives. Twenty-six percent of the alcoholic suicides had such a loss in that short space of time. The skewed distribution was again highly significant ($p < 0.01$). The original finding of a close temporal relationship between loss of a close interpersonal relationship and suicide in alcoholics had been tested as a specific hypothesis in the second study and was amply confirmed.

The nature of the interpersonal disruptions reported, in order of their frequency were: (*a*) marital separation or divorce; (*b*) breakup of an erotic relationship; (*c*) estrangement from family; and (*d*) death of a loved one. Of these, only the death of a loved one was not contributed to by the alcoholic's behavior. In keeping with their responses to the other losses, it appears that the alcoholics reacted to the finality of the loss by death in the same way as they reacted to losses of another etiology.

Because of the fact that a threatened calamity may not materialize, or that the threat may have been the product of the alcoholic's imagination, Murphy et al were careful not to count impending losses as actual losses. They do not figure in the 26 to 32% of such losses mentioned above. The confrontation described by the widow of an alcoholic suicide at the beginning of this chapter was not counted as a loss in the tabulations, for the reason that the separation had not yet occurred. The man who killed himself on the day his wife announced she was filing for divorce was also not counted as having experienced the loss of a close interpersonal relationship.

These two instances are fairly clear-cut and were described by the informants as accurately representing what was about to take place. There were other rather similar situations in which a threat of loss might be inferred. In order to avoid judgment calls, which could be subject to bias, only those events that had, in fact, taken place were counted. Counting anticipated losses might increase the vital figure by a third. What this underscores is that alcoholics are responsive both to interpersonal loss and to the threat of it. Both should be taken into account in assessing the suicidal risk presented by an acoholic patient at any given point.

The findings regarding interpersonal loss have not been subjected to replication study elsewhere, so far as the author knows. Virkkunen (10) reported failure to find evidence of a substantial frequency of recent loss preceding suicide in a series of persons characterized as "alcoholics." How the diagnosis of alcoholism was arrived at was unstated. Most importantly, the only data base was official records. There were no personal interviews with the survivors. Official records are a poor source of information for this topic, because there is no provision for systematic inquiry into the events referred to here. This cannot be regarded as a replication of Murphy's studies. It does, however, illustrate the limitations of an inquiry based entirely on official records.

Lönnqvist and Achté (11) reported conducting interviews with relatives of a series of excessive drinkers who committed suicide as well as studying official records. Their definition of "excessive drinker" was substantially broader than the authors' definition of alcoholism. It included not only persons with current symptomatic alcohol abuse, but also those with a history of periodic intoxication. Forty percent had not exhibited excessive drinking during the year preceding suicide. While those authors, like Virkkunen, report a failure to support the observations Murphy et al (8, 9) have published, it is clear that the population studied not only contained an uncertain number of alcoholics (by the author's more rigorous definition), it included a substantial number who were clearly not alcoholics. The inclusion of nonalcoholics renders this an inappropriate comparison. It was also not stated what care was exercised in inquiring about recent social disruptions. While Lönnqvist and Achté may have data that would be comparable to those of Murphy et al, they have not yet reported it in suitable form, so far as the author is aware.

If recent interpersonal loss is a stong predictor of suicide in alcoholics, it is far from infallible. Most of those alcoholics who had ever been married had experienced marital separation, if not divorce, in the past without ending their lives. What enabled them to survive such events previously, but led them to succumb on the final occasion? Some had, indeed, attempted suicide on such an earlier occasion, without fatal outcome. The question draws attention to the massive ignorance that yet surrounds the phenomenon of suicide. Few would quarrel with Beskow's (6) statement: "Suicide does not just 'happen.' It has a history." Yet that history cannot be written in generalities. It is highly individual, and probably influenced by chance as well.

A marriage might be broken with great relief at some point after it had passed through phases of intense involvement, comfort, boredom, covert and then open hostility. The disruption of another relationship might provoke both pain and despair. It was not possible under the circumstances of the author's investigations to trace the vicissitudes of these relationships over time. But the stage of the relationship might easily have been different in the eyes of the informant than in those of the partner. Whatever the stage, the disruption was clearly unwelcome to the deceased. In one case, the suicide followed by 6 weeks the beginning of a new marriage. Disruption was not reported.

Loss of autonomy, or loss of control of the relationship appeared to have been a factor in some cases. The alcoholic had previously deserted the spouse or lover, but in the final instance saw himself as deserted in turn. In other cases, there had been earlier separations, with the alcoholic always able to plead, cajole, or bully his way back into the relationship. Several widows of suicide victims reported this, along with a strong assertion that the last break had been intended to be final. One woman had not only changed her address and telephone number several times, but had finally refused to tell her family her whereabouts. Her husband had located her through them on a prior occasion. She still felt vulnerable to him if she saw him, but was unwilling to go through the trauma of a reconciliation and breakup one more time. "Yes, I'd left him before. But this time I really meant it," was the way she put it.

The element of finality was seen in another case where the separation had been of 2½ months' duration. The victim has hoped for a reconciliation with his wife, but none was in the offing even though they were in telephone contact almost daily. He paid her a visit at her invitation. Apparently the sight of a well settled apartment dashed his hopes and he killed himself a week after returning to his own abode.

An element of shame was associated with a number of the suicides. In one instance an alcoholic who had physically abused his wife throughout their marriage was now separated. He went to his wife's home and threatened her. Her son by a former marriage struck him and knocked him down, then sent him running. The young man made it clear that a return would not be tolerated. The husband seemed to regard this as the ultimate defeat. Expressions of shame or of failure were reported to have been made by a number of the suicides. In other cases, the emotion was inferred by the informant.

The finding regarding interpersonal loss, robust as it is, accounts for only a minority, albeit a large one, of alcoholic suicides. Most of the alcoholics had experienced some significant problem within the year prior to their death. While no other single type of event than interpersonal loss stood out as a frequent occurrence in relation to the suicides, disruptions of one sort or another were the rule. There were problems with health, financial problems, legal problems and others. There were also impending problems such as imminent arrest or prosecution for illegal activity, a threat of being fired, and threat of hospitalization. In contrast to depressives, whose suicides seem mainly to be a response to the internal state of depression, alcoholics appear most often to be responding to external events. That these are frequently consequences of their own behavior may or may not be important.

Another way of viewing this situation, besides looking at the prevalence of various types of occurrences, is to look at each case individually to see what the course of events was. It goes without saying that each case was unique, and the author plans to present all the details at another time. Approaching the problem from the viewpoint that alcoholics who take their lives may be reacting to the external world, a judgment is made in each case as to the most likely precipitant of self-destruction. Table 6.1 lists the author's personal conclusions in this matter.

While interpersonal disruptions comprise the single most common class of presumed precipitating events, they were still in the minority. The variety of external events thought to have precipitated suicide was quite broad. Several victims had been living on savings or inheritance and killed themselves when the money ran out. Threat of rehospitalization was the immediate precipitant in at least two instances. News of a severe medical illness—cancer, multiple myeloma, necessity for amputation of a hand—had immediately preceded three suicides. Loss of a good job, marked reduction in employment status, and trouble with the law figured as precipitants in more than

Table 6.1. Most Important Reason for Suicide

Reason	No.
Marital separation/divorce	8
Friction with spouse/lover	9
Expectation of loss (realistic)	5
Estrangement from family	2
Bereavement	2
Friction with family	1
Job trouble	4
Financial trouble	3
Trouble with the law	2
Depressed (as principal or only reason)	6
Feeling of disgrace	2
Feared rehospitalization	2
Inability to control drinking	1
Other	2
No provocation identified	1
	50

one case. A majority had experienced serious trouble related to employment during the year preceding death.

Owing to the close association between depressive disorder and suicide and, also, its association with alcoholism, it might be expected that alcoholics who take their lives would be recognized to be depressed as well. While this was true in over three-quarters of the cases, 22% of the alcoholics who took their lives had not exhibited the syndrome of depressive disorder (Table 6.2). From the degree of closeness of the informant to the victim and his or her knowledge of the behavior and state of mind of the victim, this finding does not appear to be a function of a lack of information. It suggests that while many alcoholics who take their lives are depressed at the time, a substantial minority are not. The presence of depression was not found to be related to the presence of interpersonal loss. On the other hand, in seven cases, environmental precipitants were not identified, and it appeared that a deepening depression was the primary cause of the suicide in six of them (Table 6.1).

The implications of the findings reported here seem fairly clear-cut. Murphy et al found no former alcoholics among their suicides, only active ones. While it is possible that this is an artifact of reporting, it would appear that successful treatment of alcoholism, resulting in prolonged sobriety, would be a substantial preventive measure. Since one-third of the alcoholics in Murphy and Robins' 1957 study (9) and half of those in the replication study (8) had seen a physician within 1 month of their death, this is clearly a clinical problem. For active alcoholics under medical care, alertness to the vicissitudes of the patient's life is important. Impending or very recent major disruptions should be a signal for increased emotional and environmental support. This might come in the form of protective hospitalization, more frequent physician contact, or finding family members or friends who are willing to provide additional emotional support in these times of crisis. The lifetime risk of suicide in alcoholism is approximately the same as for major depressive disorder, around 15%. This figure might be reduced by effective treatment of the alcoholism and by special attention at times of life crisis.

Table 6.2. Clinical Diagnoses and Affectional Loss Experience of 50 Alcoholic Suicides*

	No. (%) of Total (N = 50)	% Having Loss within	
		6 Weeks	1 Year
Uncomplicated alcoholism	11 (22)	45	64
Alcoholism and secondary affective disorder	24 (48)	21	67
Alcoholism, secondary affective disorder, and other†	4 (8)	25	75
Alcoholism and possible secondary affective disorder	4 (8)	0	25
Alcoholism and other‡	3 (6)	33	33
Primary affective disorder with secondary alcoholism	4 (8)	25	50

*From Murphy GE, Armstrong JW Jr, Hermele SL, Fischer JR, Clendenin WW: Suicide and alcoholism. Interpersonal loss confirmed as a predictor. *Arch Gen Psychiatry* 36:65–69, 1979. Copyright 1979, American Medical Association.
† Organic brain syndrome, two; anxiety neurosis, one; sexual deviation, one.
‡ Schizophrenia and mental deficiency, one; paranoia, one; narcotic addiction (by history), one.

96 / *Suicide*

In the time since the studies reported here were done, substance abuse other than alcohol has attained a prominence previously unthought of. To the extent that dependence on one substance is psychologically like dependence on another, it may be that substance abusers of various kinds may be found to partake of the same characteristics as alcoholics, including heightened reactivity to life events. Until hard data are forthcoming, it may be wise to consider all substance abusers at risk of suicide when the circumstances of their lives are strikingly disrupted.

References

1. American Psychiatric Association: *Diagnostic and Statistical Manual of Mental Disorders*, ed 3. Washington, DC, American Psychiatric Association, 1980.
2. Feighner JP, Robins E, Guze SB, Woodruff RA, Winokur G, Munoz R: Diagnostic criteria for use in psychiatric research. *Arch Gen Psychiatry* 26:57–63, 1972.
3. Robins E, Murphy GE, Wilkinson RH Jr, Gassner S, Kayes J: Some clinical considerations in the prevention of suicide based on a study of 134 successful suicides. *Am J Public Health* 49:888–899, 1959.
4. Dorpat TL, Ripley HS: A study of suicide in the Seattle area. *Compr Psychiatry* 1:349–359, 1960.
5. Barraclough B, Bunch J, Nelson B, Sainsbury P: A hundred cases of suicide: clinical aspects. *Br J Psychiatry* 125:355–373, 1974.
6. Beskow J: Suicide and mental disorder in Swedish men. *Acta Psychiatr Scand (Suppl)* 277:1–138, 1979.
7. Chynoweth R, Tonge JI, Armstrong J: Suicide in Brisbane—a retrospective psychosocial study. *Aust NZ J Psychiatry* 14:37–45, 1980.
8. Murphy GE, Armstrong JW Jr, Hermele SL, Fischer JR, Clendenin WW: Suicide and Alcoholism. Interpersonal loss confirmed as a predictor. *Arch Gen Psychiatry* 36:65–69, 1979.
9. Murphy GE, Robins E: Social factors in suicide. *JAMA* 199:303–308, 1967.
10. Virkkunen M: Alcoholism and suicides in Helsinki. *Psychiatr Feen*, pp 201–207, 1971.
11. Lönnqvist J, Achté KA: Excessive drinking in psychiatric patients who later committed suicide. *Psychiatr Fenn*, pp 209–213, 1971.

7

Suicide in Schizophrenia

Alec Roy, M.B., B.Chir., M.R.C.P., M.R.C.Psych.

Bleuler (1) described the suicidal drive as "the most serious of schizophrenic symptoms," and a number of follow-up studies over a period of 45 years have all found that schizophrenic illness carries with it an increased risk of suicide (Table 7.1). Miles (6) in 1977 reviewed all available follow-up studies and estimated that 10% of schizophrenics die by suicide and that in the United States approximately 3800 schizophrenics commit suicide each year.

There are large variations between studies for the calculated suicide risk. Using the records of the Houston Veterans Administration Hospital, Pokorny (7) in 1964 calculated that the suicide rate for male schizophrenic patients was 167/100,000/year compared with the then US national rate of about 10/100,000/year. More recently, in 1982, from the Missouri psychiatric case register, Evenson et al (8) estimated that the age-adjusted suicide rate for male schizophrenic patients was 210/100,000, and the rate for females was 90/100,000. Also in 1982 Wilkinson (9), using the Camberwell Psychiatric Case Register, estimated that the annual rate of suicide for first-admission schizophrenic patients was between 500 and 750/100,000.

Another source of information about suicide in schizophrenia comes from reported series of psychiatric patients known to have committed suicide. In such series schizophrenic patients usually account for up to a third or more of patients (10–13).

The social and psychiatric factors thought to be associated with suicide in schizophrenic patients will be reviewed in this chapter.

AGE

Individuals in the general population who commit suicide tend to be middle-aged or elderly (14, 15), whereas psychiatric patients who kill themselves are increasingly young (12). Eastwood and Peacocke (16) noted that this is particularly true for schizophrenic patients. Since 1980 there have been six studies of schizophrenic patients known to have committed suicide. The mean age of the total 161 patients in these studies was 33.1 years (Table 7.2).

There are three studies showing that schizophrenic patient suicides tend to be younger than other psychiatric patients. Breier and Astrachan (19) found them to be younger than other psychiatric patient controls—means of 30.3 and 43.7 years ($p < 0.01$). Langley and Bayatti (22) reported that male schizophrenic patient suicides were younger than male depressed suicides—means of 31 and 52 years ($p < 0.001$). Virkkunen's (23) schizophrenia and paranoid psychosis patient suicides were younger than nonschizophrenic patient suicides—means of 39.4 and 43.4 years.

Table 7.1. Suicide in Follow-up Studies of Schizophrenic Patients

Author	Location	No. of Patients	Length of Follow-up (Years)	% Who Committed Suicide
Rennie, 1939 (2)	Johns Hopkins	500	20	11
Markowe et al, 1967 (3)	England	100	10	6
Winokur and Tsuang, 1975 (4)	Iowa	170	40	10
McGlashan, 1984 (5)	Chestnut Lodge	163	14.8	8
Roy et al, 1986 (85)	National Institute of Mental Health	100	4.5	6

Table 7.2. Age and Sex Ratio in Studies of Chronic Schizophrenic Patient Suicides Reported Since 1980*

Author	No. of Patients	Mean Age (Years)	% Male
Cheng, 1982 (unpublished data)	12	31.0	83.3
Roy, 1982 (17)	30	27.9	80
Hogan and Awad, 1983 (18)	67	35.5	80.6
Breier and Astrachan, 1984 (19)	20	30.3	90
Drake et al., 1984 (20)	15	31.7	60
Wilkinson and Bacon, 1985 (21)	17	42	47

* None of these studies was from a Veterans Administration hospital.

SEX

A number of studies from different countries have suggested that male schizophrenic patients seem to be more at risk for suicide than females (24, 25). In the United States, Rennie's follow-up study (2) showed that 63.6% of the schizophrenic patient suicides were male. In Breier and Astrachan's New Haven study (19) 90% of the 20 suicides were male, and the suicide group contained significantly more males than a randomly selected control group of 81 living schizophrenic patients. In the Iowa 500 follow-up study (26) the suicide risk was raised for male, but not female, schizophrenic patients, and in New York state deinstitutionalized male, but not female, schizophrenic patients were found to have an increased risk of death—particularly from accidents and suicide (27).

In Canada, 13 of 16 schizophrenic patients (81.2%) who committed suicide in Montreal were male (28). In Finland, Virkkunen found that 50 of 82 (61%) schizophrenic and paranoid psychosis patient suicides were male (23). From Norway, Noreik (29) reported that 15 of 524 male schizophrenic patients (2.9%) committed suicide in the first 5 years of follow-up, compared with only 1 of 399 females (0.25%) ($p < 0.001$). In the six studies reported since 1980, 73.5% of the schizophrenic patient suicides were male (Table 7.2).

This trend toward a preponderance of male schizophrenic suicides may partly be nonspecific, as males in general tend to commit suicide more than females (8, 15, 30). What is of note is that among suicides in the general population the male to female sex ratio is about 3 to 1 (and this ratio is probably less among psychiatric patients (8)), while in three recent series of schizophrenic patient suicides males outnumber females about 4 to 1 (17, 19, 20). This male preponderance may partly reflect the fact that the age of onset of schizophrenia is approximately 5 years earlier in males than in females (31–33): about 9 of 10 male patients, compared to only 2 of 3 females, become schizophrenic before 30 years of age (31). For example, in Roy's study (17), male suicides had begun their illness at a significantly earlier age than females (mean 21.0 versus 26.4 years, $p < 0.01$) and in the study of Drake and co-workers (20) male suicides also had a significantly younger onset of illness than females (mean 21.6 versus 26.0 years, $p < 0.05$). However, recently Leventhal et al (34) found that both schizophrenic and nonschizophrenic male patients reported their psychiatric symptoms earlier than females. They suggested that males are perceived and dealt with by others in a different fashion than females; males are expected to assume responsibility in social and financial matters earlier than females.

A recent Finnish study also suggests that schizophrenia may affect the sexes differently. Salokangas (35) followed 175 schizophrenic patients a mean 8 years after their first admission and found that there were only small differences in psychiatric symptoms between the sexes but that social, psychosexual, and work adjustments were poorer in male patients than in female patients. More of the women were married, and more of the men were living with parents. In their premorbid psychosexual development, significantly more male than female patients had never had a social relationship with the opposite sex. Salokangas concluded that the social withdrawal associated with schizophrenia affects the male social role, which he believes involves greater activity and the need to demonstrate competence, considerably more adversely than it does the female role.

MARITAL STATUS

Suicide rates in general are higher among those who are single, divorced, or widowed than they are among the married (14). Schizophrenia occurs mainly in young adults, the majority of schizophrenic patients are unmarried, and schizophrenic patient suicides tend to be unmarried. Cohen and co-workers (36) found that although 57.5% of the schizophrenic patient suicides in their series were unmarried, there were no significant differences for marital status when compared to living schizophrenic patient controls. Similarly, Hogan and Awad (18) found that although 60 of 67 schizophrenic patient suicides (89.6%) were unmarried, so were exactly the same number of matched schizophrenic controls; and in Drake and co-workers' series (20) 100% of the suicides were unmarried, as were 93% of the schizophrenic controls.

Breier and Astrachan (19) reported that 18 of 20 suicides (90%) were unmarried, as were 71 of the 81 (87.7%) control schizophrenics, but significantly more of the suicides had never been married when compared with 18 nonschizophrenic patient suicides (70% versus 28%, $p < 0.05$). In Roy's study (17), although there were no significant differences for marital status, 83% of suicides and 70% of controls were single, there was a sex difference among the suicides as significantly more females than males were married or divorced. Whether the explanation for the previously discussed earlier age of onset of schizophrenia in males is cultural or biological, being unmarried is a risk factor for suicide in psychiatric patients (12). Thus, because more male than female schizophrenic patients are unmarried (31), their single status represents a suicide risk factor, particularly for male schizophrenics.

WHEN IN THEIR ILLNESS DO THEY COMMIT SUICIDE?

Although an excessive mortality from "unnatural" causes has been found among men with acute schizophrenia (37), in the majority of series schizophrenic patients who commit suicide have suffered from chronic schizophrenia. Yarden (38), for example, reported that all 20 schizophrenic suicides known to the Jacobi Unit of the Bronx State Hospital during the first 5 years of its community program were chronic schizophrenics. No patient committed suicide in the year after his or her first admission. In the Iowa 500 follow-up study the schizophrenic patients who committed suicide had chronic schizophrenia and committed suicide during the first few years of the 40-year follow-up period. In Roy's study (17) the male patients committed suicide after a mean 4.8 years of illness and the females after 9.8 years. Similarly the patients in Breier and Astrachan's study (19) committed suicide after an average 7.8 years of illness, those in the series of Drake and co-workers (20) after a mean 8.4 years, the patients in L Cheng's series (unpublished data) after a mean 7 years, and those reported by Wilkinson and Bacon (21) after a mean 10 years of illness.

WHEN IN THEIR PSYCHIATRIC CARE DO THEY COMMIT SUICIDE?

Schizophrenic patients tend to commit suicide around their last hospitalization. Copas and Robin (39) examined psychiatric inpatient suicides occurring in England and Wales and found that the suicide risk was highest for both sexes in the first week of admission and that after 3 to 5 years as an inpatient the suicide risk was no greater than the risk in the general population. They also found that the suicide risk for affective disorder inpatients was only 1½ times that of schizophrenic inpatients. Watkins and co-workers (40) reviewed the diagnoses in four studies of suicide among psychiatric inpatients and found that schizophrenic patients accounted for 87 of the total 194 suicides

In most studies a minority of schizophrenic patient suicides have occurred during hospitalization. The great majority of these do not occur in the hospital ward but in the grounds or in the community when the patient is on a pass, weekend leave, or absent without leave (41). Among outpatients who commit suicide a time of increased risk is the period after discharge from the last hospitalization (9, 42, 43). Most studies reveal that up to 50% of schizophrenic patient suicides occur in the first few weeks and months after discharge (Table 7.3). Why the postdischarge period is one of increased risk will be discussed below.

Table 7.3. When in Their Care Do Chronic Schizophrenic Patients Commit Suicide?

Author	No. of Patients	Suicide	
		As Inpatient	After Discharge
Cohen et al, 1964 (36)	40	18 (45%)	22 (55%) on pass, absent without leave, trial visit or recent discharge
Pokorny, 1964 (7)	31	2 (6.5%)	15 (48.4%) within 1 month
Warnes, 1968 (28)	16	8 (50%)	8 (50%) soon after discharge
Yarden, 1974 (38)	20	2 (10%)	11 (55%) within 3 months
Roy, 1982 (17)	30	7 (23.3%)	13 (43.3%) within 6 months
Drake et al, 1984 (20)	15	5 (33.3%)	7 (46.7%) within 6 months
Wilkinson and Bacon, 1958 (21)	17	6 (35.3%)	Mean 10.5 months for females and 32 months for males

METHOD OF SUICIDE

In general males tend to commit suicide using active violent methods like jumping, shooting, hanging, or stabbing, while females tend to use passive methods like drug overdosage or drowning (44). In Toronto 7 of 24 male schizophrenic patient suicides threw themselves under a subway train, 8 shot themselves, and 6 jumped from high buildings; 2 of the 3 patients who overdosed were female (17). In Breier and Astrachan's study 14 of 18 male suicides used highly lethal active suicide methods; 7 of the 14 used firearms. Yarden also noted that his schizophrenic "patients choose easily available methods": 30% jumped, 30% overdosed, 3 hung themselves, 2 went under a subway train, and 1 shot himself. Schizophrenic outpatients tend to be unemployed and have little money (17), which may partly determine their method of committing suicide.

Watkins and co-workers (40) found that unusual suicide methods used in the hospital were head ramming, asphyxia by the aspiration of paper or food, and exsanguination by tearing blood vessels with fingers, and they noted that these methods are constantly available to schizophrenic inpatients and that the seclusion room may provide an ideal opportunity to try them.

PREVIOUS SUICIDE ATTEMPT

A large percentage of schizophrenic patients attempt suicide. Planasky and Johnson (45) reported that suicidal ideas and attempts were found in half of a sample of 205 schizophrenic male patients, and Roy et al found that 55% of 127 schizophrenic patients had attempted suicide during a mean 6 years of illness (46). Similarly a past suicide attempt has been made by a large percentage of schizophrenic patients who eventually commit suicide (Table 7.4).

A previous suicide attempt is generally considered to be an indicator of increased risk of eventually committing suicide (47, 48). Wilkinson and Bacon (21) found that of 124 first-ever schizophrenic parasuicides, 10 (8%) committed suicide over the subsequent years and that this percentage was similar to the 1% per annum of nonschizophrenic parasuicides who might be expected eventually to commit suicide. Shaffer and co-workers (49) found that a previous suicide attempt had been recorded in the case histories of significantly more schizophrenic patients who subsequently committed suicide than schizophrenic controls and that the number of previous attempts was the most important single variable associated with eventual suicide. The

Table 7.4. Previous Suicide Attempt in Chronic Schizophrenic Patients Who Committed Suicide

Author	No. of Suicides	No. (%) Who Made Previous Suicide Attempt
Cohen et al, 1964 (36)	40	22 (55%)
Warnes, 1968 (28)	16	6 (37.5%)
Yarden, 1974 (38)	20	13 (65%)
Shaffer et al, 1974 (49)	12	5 (42%)
Virkkunen, 1974 (23)	82	39 (47.6%)
Cheng, 1982 (unpublished data)	12	7 (58.3%)
Roy, 1982 (17)	30	12 (40%)
Breier and Astrachan, 1984 (19)	20	12 (60%)
Drake et al, 1984 (20)	15	11 (73%)

20 suicides in Breier and Astrachan's study had made significantly more prior attempts than a sex-matched control group of 20 living schizophrenic patients. In the Chestnut Lodge follow-up study (50) there was also a trend for the 13 schizophrenic suicides to have made a prior suicide threat or attempt more frequently than 150 schizophrenic patients who had not committed suicide.

However, although 12 of 30 suicides (40%) in Roy's series (17) had attempted suicide there was no significant difference compared with 30 living schizophrenic controls, 11 of whom had attempted suicide (37%). Similarly, Drake and co-workers (20) reported that although 73% of 15 schizophrenic patient suicides had made an earlier attempt, there was no significant difference compared with living schizophrenic controls, 49% of whom had attempted suicide. Thus, at this time the 1961 conclusion of Fareberow and co-workers (51) still seems to be appropriate. They found that 40% of their schizophrenic controls had a past history of a suicide attempt or ideation, "indicating that simply knowing this fact is not an accurate indicator of suicide in a schizophrenic group."

DEPRESSION

Depression is closely associated with suicide in schizophrenic patients. In studies over the last 30 years depressive symptoms have been reported in the last period of psychiatric contact in a substantial percentage of schizophrenic patient suicides (Table 7.5).

Warnes (28) reported that 12 of 16 schizophrenic patient suicides (75%) had a "hopeless awareness of their own pathology," and 4 (25%) had been treated with antidepressants or electroconvulsive treatment. Yarden (38), as well as examining the case records, also interviewed therapists, family members, social workers and others. He reported the psychiatric symptoms registered in the 3 months before the patient's suicide: "The communication of hopelessness and despair in the form of sad comments or gloomy predictions was common to 65% of the patients. Direct verbal suicidal statements were made by 50%." Anorexia and weight loss were found in 80% and motor retardation in 45% of the patients. Virkkunen (23) also interviewed at least one informant and found that 57 of the 82 (69.5%) patient suicides in his series were "depressed before committing suicide." Hogan and Awad (18) compared patterns of drug prescribing and found that significantly more of 67 schizophrenic patient suicides were receiving antidepressant medications than were schizophrenic controls.

In Roy's study (17) significantly more of the schizophrenic patient suicides than

Table 7.5. Depression in Chronic Schizophrenic Patients Who Committed Suicide

Author	No. of Suicides	No. (%) Who Had Depression
Levy and Southcombe, 1953 (52)	23	6 (25.2%)
Beisser and Blanchette, 1961 (53)	32	"High frequency of depression"
Cohen et al, 1964 (36)	40	28 (70%)
Warnes, 1968 (28)	16	12 (75%)
Yarden, 1974 (38)	20	13 (65%)
Virkkunen, 1974 (23)	82	57 (69.5%)
Cheng, 1982 (unpublished data)	12	12 (100%)
Roy, 1982 (17)	30	16 (53.3%)
Drake et al, 1984 (20)	15	12 (80%)

controls had in the past both been diagnosed as suffering from a depressive episode and been treated for depression with either antidepressant medication or electroconvulsive treatment: 17 of the 30 suicides (56.6%) had had a past depressive episode, and 14 (46.6%) had received antidepressant medication or electroconvulsive treatment. Also in their last period of psychiatric contact significantly more of the suicides were recorded as having associated depressive symptoms, which were present in 16 (53.3%). Their last admission had been precipitated by accompanying depressive symptoms and/or suicidal ideas or impulses—significantly more than in the schizophrenic controls ($p < 0.02$). Wilkinson and Bacon (21) also found that in about half of the suicides in their series the last admission had been for a mixture of schizophrenic and depressive symptomatology.

STRESS AND LIFE EVENTS

Many psychiatric patient suicides have recently experienced stress and life events (42, 54–56), and suicide attempters report 4 times as many life events as controls (57). Fareberow and co-workers (50) performed psychological autopsies for each of 30 schizophrenic patient suicides. They concluded that they "were, by and large, persons who felt under stress." "It can be said that . . . suicide resulted when they found themselves in a stressful situation from which they saw no other means of escape." Yarden noted that his schizophrenic suicides became depressed and suicidal "often following the disruption of various interpersonal relations or existential conditions on which the patient depended. These included marital abandonment, actual or threatened separation from parents, being jilted by boyfriend, rehospitalization, discharge from hospital, loss of job, or dropping out from ambitious rehabilitation or reeducation programs."

However, Breier and Astrachan reported that schizophrenic patient suicides had experienced significantly less life events than nonschizophrenic patient suicides. But, they did not use living schizophrenic controls and they retrospectively reconstructed life events. Interestingly, the most common life event experienced by the schizophrenic suicides was to be told that they could no longer return to live with their family. Discharge from the hospital may involve the loss of supportive relationships with nurses, co-patients, and others. Life events involving losses are known to be associated with the onset of depression (58). A recent study demonstrated that depressed schizophrenic patients, compared to nondepressed schizophrenic controls, had experienced more life events—and more undesirable life events—in the 6 months before the onset of depressive symptoms (59).

SEVERITY OF ILLNESS

There is some evidence that the nature of the schizophrenic illness may be a determinant of suicide. In Roy's study significantly more suicides than controls had a severe relapsing illness; the male suicides had a mean 4.1 admissions during 4.8 years of illness—almost one admission each year. Yarden in 1974 (38) reported similar findings: "most had a rather chronic course with periodic exacerbations and remissions and with numerous discharges and readmissions." In the 5 years before suicide his patients had a mean of 10 admissions—an average of 2 admissions a year—and had spent a total of 26.4 of their last 60 months in hospital. In the 2-year period before suicide these 20 patients had an average of 6 admissions—a mean of 3 a year—and had spent a mean 8.1 of their last 24 months in hospital. A recent 6-year follow-up study (60) found that an unexpectedly large number of schizophrenic patients initially diagnosed as having a poor prognosis illness had died as a result of suicide or probable suicide.

ADEQUACY OF TREATMENT

As most acts of suicide are theoretically amenable to prevention, it might be thought that schizophrenic patients who commit suicide have not received adequate treatment. However, there is little in the literature to support this. Cohen and co-workers (36) found no significant difference between schizophrenic patient suicide and control groups for treatment with chlorpromazine. Twenty-six of the 30 suicides in Roy's study (17) were receiving adequate regular neuroleptic medication, as were 60 of the 67 reported by Hogan and Awad (18) and 9 of the 15 reported by Drake and co-workers (20). Yarden (38) also found that his suicides "were treated adequately with psychopharmacological medications. At the time of their suicides, all were on a regime of phenothiazines or similar antipsychotics in moderate to high doses, and most also received tricyclic antidepressants."

There is also little in the literature to support the notion that schizophrenic patients who commit suicide have received inadequate nonpsychopharmacological treatment during their last hospitalization. For example, in Roy's study there were no significant differences between the suicide and control groups for the mean duration of their last admission, the numbers receiving social case work, vocational rehabilitation assessment, or day care treatment after the last admission. Nor were there any significant differences for the frequency of subsequent outpatient appointments. Drake and co-workers (20) also found that no treatment variables were associated with suicide. However, Fareberow and co-workers (51) noted that not enough of the suicide patients in their series had received a meaningful evaluation for individual or group psychotherapy. This might have allowed for a continuing supportive relationship after discharge. They also noted that none of the milieu therapies appeared to improve the patients' ability to make a better adjustment outside of hospital.

There are, however, recent studies that demonstrate that the care that schizophrenic patients receive in the community is often inadequate. Caton and co-workers (61) studied the discharge planning process on 119 schizophrenic patients in New York. They found that the staff were most successful in planning drug treatment and aftercare and least successful in planing living arrangements in the community. In 39% of the patients the discharge planners recommended a change in the current living arrangements but an alternative was found for only 13% of those in need, largely because of a lack of such options as halfway houses, shared apartments, and other supervised living settings. Although the discharge planners assessed that 55% of the patients were in need of vocational rehabilitation, this was arranged for only a third—nonreferral was due to patient refusal, poor motivation, or severe disability.

Caton and co-workers (61) found that effective discharge planning successfully connected the patients to community treatment services and resulted in better patient compliance and tenure in the community, but poor discharge planning resulted in inadequate linkage to community services and early rehospitalization. In a recent follow-up study of schizophrenic patients in England, Johnstone and co-workers (62) also found that severe emotional, social, and financial difficulties were commonplace; 27% of the sample had no contact with medical or social services, a further 14% saw only community nurses, and 24% saw only their general practioners. In Scotland, McCreadie and co-workers (63) found that the occupational activity of more than a third of schizophrenic patients attending care was inappropriate.

NEUROLEPTIC MEDICATION

The possible role of neuroleptics in depression and suicide in schizophrenic patients has been controversial. It has been claimed that neuroleptics, particularly depot preparations, cause depression, and occasionally suicide, in schizophrenic patients (64). However, although depression in schizophrenic patients is common (65–67) it now seems unlikely that neuroleptics play much part in the etiology (68). Warnes (28) compared the phenothiazine dosage in 16 schizophrenic patient suicides with that in 16 schizophrenic patients who had shown past suicidal behavior and in fact found that "significantly more control subjects were on a higher dosage than the experimental group." Cohen et al (36) found no significant difference between schizophrenic patient suicides and controls for the daily dosage of chlorpromazine; in both groups the mean daily dosage was over 300 mg.

In Roy's study (17) there was no significant difference between suicide and control groups, when all neuroleptics were converted to daily chlorpromazine equivalent dosages—means of 654.0 mg and 742.3 mg, respectively. Hogan and Awad (18) matched 67 suicides with schizophrenic patient controls and also found no significant difference for drug dosage—mean equivalent chlorpromazine daily doses of 688 mg and 758 mg, respectively (doses very similar to those found in Roy's study); 20 patients in each group were receiving depot fluphenazine. However, they did find that the 16 suicides, compared to the 11 controls, who were being treated with fluphenazine enanthate injections were receiving a higher dose. They speculated that these patients may have been more severly ill and thus needed a higher dose.

Also Wilkinson and Bacon (21) found no difference between schizophrenic patient suicide and control groups for the proportions receiving depot or oral neuroleptics. Shear et al (69) reported two psychotic male patients who developed severe akathisia while receiving depot fluphenazine and who both committed suicide by jumping. Although the authors were not sure that the akathisia caused the deaths, they thought that the akathisia probably was the immediate precipitant of suicide.

HALLUCINATIONS AND DELUSIONS

Some clinicians will know of a patient who committed suicide because of auditory hallucinations instructing him to "kill yourself." Some textbooks emphasize the importance of instructing hallucinations in assessing the suicidal risk in schizophrenic patients (70). However, this is probably an infrequent cause of suicide.

Lehmann and Ban (71) found no significant relationship between suicidal thoughts, threats, or attempts and hallucinations in schizophrenic patients. In Roy's study (17) in only 2 of the 30 suicides was it reasonably certain that the patient had committed suicide as a consequence of instructing hallucinations (1 by jumping and 1 by hanging), and there was no significant difference compared to the 30 living schizophrenic controls, 2 of who had attempted suicide following instructing hallucinations. Similarly, Breier and Astrachan (19) found that none of the 20 suicides in their series could be attributed to hallucinated suicidal commands, Drake and co-workers (20) reported that none of 15 suicides had command hallucinations, and Wilkinson and Bacon (21) found no difference between schizophrenic patient suicide and control groups for a history of auditory hallucinations.

Other clinicians may know of patients who killed themselves to escape persecutory delusions, i.e., "I am going to kill myself before letting the Mafia (or CIA) torture me and kill me." However, Farberow and co-workers (51) found that "although ordinarily the words schizophrenic suicide conjure up the image of a psychotic person who might kill himself in response to a hallucinated command, delusional impulse or a derelistic thought ... suicide occurred in almost all cases where there was some evidence of improved organization and control in the patient." "There was no doubt that these patients had improved with tranquilizing drugs so they were no longer so highly disturbed as they had been on admission and were in a fairly good contact with reality." Similarly, Yarden (38) noted that 13 of 20 schizophrenic patients committed suicide when either in remission or in a chronic defect state and that "features of florid psychotic activity and lack of impulse control were characteristic only of some of the patients." Breier and Astrachan (19) found that only 3 of 20 suicides were in an exacerbated, disorganized psychotic state at the time of death; L Cheng (unpublished data) found that only 1 of 12 suicides could be considered to be due to delusions; and Drake and co-workers (20) found that none of their 15 suicides had persecutory delusions.

Before neuroleptics were discovered Kraepelin (72) observed that "... suicide, especially in the first period of the malady, is not infrequent and occurs, sometimes without any recognizable cause, also in patients who for long have been weak-minded and apparently quiet." Suicide is generally considered to be a multidetermined act (73). It is therefore likely that, when present, command hallucinations or persecutory delusions may play an indirect part in a suicide by contributing to the development of feelings of helplessness and hopelessness. Some support for this formulation comes from a recent study of psychotic children in which significantly more of those with auditory hallucinations, compared to those without, had associated affective symptoms (74).

SOCIAL ISOLATION

Social isolation has repeatedly been found to be frequent among suicides in both the general population and psychiatric patients (12, 14). Many schizophrenic patients on leaving hospital face social isolation, and this may play a contributory role in their committing suicide. In Roy's study (17) 90% of the suicides were unmarried, 80% were unemployed, and 46.6% lived alone; and in Breier and Astrachan's study (19) 90% were unmarried, 80% were unemployed, and 30% lived alone. In Yarden's series (38) 70% of the suicide patients were unemployed and 25% lived alone; and in the series of Drake and co-workers (20) 100% were unmarried, 93% were unemployed and 60% lived alone.

Being unmarried, unemployed, and living alone may lead to social isolation. In Roy's study (17) the young male suicide patients had a mean age of 25.8 years and over the previous mean 4.8 years had had almost one hospital admission each year. Their chronic illness, and the repeated hospital admissions which it had caused, greatly undermined their educational and occupational goals as well as their heterosexual adjustment and thus contributed to their social isolation. Social isolation is particularly unfortunate for schizophrenic patients. Breier and Strauss (75), studying psychotic patients over the 12-month period after hospitalization, described the positive and helpful effect that social relationships may have for such patients while they are attempting to readjust and rebuild their lives. Wilson (76) found that among 17 psychiatric patient suicides (two-thirds of whom were schizophrenic) only a quarter were engaged in either a meaningful or therapeutic relationship with at least one other person.

WHY DO THEY COMMIT SUICIDE?

Schizophrenic patients who commit suicide do not form a homogeneous group. There are probably several types of suicidal motivation. However, the majority are male and are relatively young. It is likely that the chronic difficulties, unemployment, and social isolation that they face—in addition to having to cope with the symptoms of their schizophrenic illness—may lead some patients to feel helpless, hopeless, and depressed and to develop suicidal ideas which they eventually act on.

Virkkunen (23) interviewed relatives and aquaintances and found that 57 of the 82 (69.5%) schizophrenic and paranoid patients in his series were depressed before committing suicide and that 37 (45.1%) expressed suicidal threats or thoughts prior to committing suicide. Twenty of the 57 patients (24.4%) had been depressed for a month or more, and 37 (45.1%) were depressed immediately before suicide; the average duration of depression was 1½ months. The informants thought that there was an apparent rational reason for committing suicide in 64.9% of these depressed schizophrenic patients. These included the hopeless nature of the illness, work problems or inability to find work, death, divorce, other interpersonal losses, hospitalization denied, or loneliness. In 50 of the 82 patients (61%) the informants thought that the suicide was premeditated and that the fear of becoming a chronic inpatient was present in 32 of them (39%), while 62 (75.6%) did not believe that psychiatric treatment would be helpful to them anymore.

Virkkunen (77) also sent a questionnaire to the doctors and psychiatric personnel concerned with the subgroups of schizophrenic and nonschizophrenic patient controls who had been in treatment before committing suicide, inquiring about the patients' attitudes toward both treatment and the hospital personnel during the 2 months before suicide. Significantly more schizophrenic than control suicides had an indifferent or negative attitude toward the psychiatric personnel, including the doctor (60% versus 27.5%). Both the doctors and other personnel also rated significantly more of the schizophrenic suicides as having ceased to request support or attention (67.5% versus 45%) and that in significantly more of them their attitude toward medication had become at least partly negative (45% versus 10%). Virkkunen interpreted these findings as further evidence that in schizophrenic patients a state of despair often predominates before suicide and may manifest itself in negative attitudes toward personnel and treatment.

Similarly Fareberow and co-workers (51) noted that in some suicide patients "Statements such as 'nothing is being done for me,' 'other people don't like me,' 'I should end it all,' and 'there's no place for me anywhere' were frequent . . . ." Cheng (unpublished data) noted that his suicides had depressive "thoughts about the future. 'Will I ever live a normal life again?' 'Life is pointless.'" Fareberow and co-workers noted that some suicides "knew they were ill, and depended on the hospital for protection." Others manifested "severe feelings of inadequacy, lack of personal worth, or guilt."

Bleuler (1) observed: "People are being forced to live a life that has become unbearable for them for valid reasons." Fareberow and co-workers noted that "in almost all the 30 schizophrenic suicides studied, the suicide was a somewhat organized and planned action by the patient in an apparent effort to extricate himself from his intolerable life situation, from which he could see no other way out." Baechler (78) considered that "schizophrenics do not kill themselves insofar as they are schizophrenic but insofar as they are persons who know they are schizophrenic or are threatened with becoming so and who wish to avoid this fated outcome."

Drake and co-workers (20) found that significantly more of their schizophrenic suicides, compared to controls, had a college education. They drew attention to the inability of educated patients, with high performance expectations, to accept the declining functional ability that schizophrenia may cause. Significantly more of their suicides than controls, at their last hospital admission also had a fear of mental disintegration. Their last admission was to a public mental hospital, and Drake and co-workers were impressed by the downward drift of these suicides and the painful awareness that they had about their illness. Similarly, in the Chestnut Lodge follow-up study (50) the schizophrenic suicides had displayed superior premorbid functioning and demonstrated greater retention of their ability to think abstractly and conceptually than the schizophrenic patients who did not commit suicide. Cheng (unpublished data) noted that all 12 schizophrenic suicides in his mental hospital series had at least a grade 12 education and several had some higher education. Intelligent, ambitious, young males who develop schizophrenia may be more likely to become despondent, hopeless, and depressed, and then be at risk to commit suicide because of insight into the reality that they may never be able to achieve the expectations that they had for themselves.

THE POSTDISCHARGE PERIOD

Studies indicate that the period after discharge from a psychiatric admission is a period of increased risk for suicide. Temoche et al (79) estimated that among psychiatric patients in general this risk is 34 times as great as the risk in the general population. Winokur (80) calculated that in the first 3 months after hospitalization the suicide rate for male psychiatric patients in Iowa was 70 times as high as that for all Iowa males.

Bolin and co-workers (54) reported that two-thirds of a series of 27 patients—12 of whom were schizophrenic—who committed suicide while on home leave from a mental hospital had experienced "real, threatened or imagined loss in the previous six months" involving spouse, home, job, children, money, love, etc. Pokorny and Kaplan (42) matched 20 male Veterans Administration inpatients known to have committed suicide after discharge with controls for age, race, and time at risk in the community. A defenselessness score was obtained by summing scores on seven items on the Brief Psychiatric Rating Scale completed at the time of last admission. Life events were inquired about from informants who knew the suicides, and directly from controls, using the Social Readjustment Rating Scale of Holmes and Rahe. Adverse life events were consensually judged by three raters. Significantly more suicides than controls were distributed into the "high defenselessness—one or more adverse life events" category than into any of the other three possible categories. The "defenselessness" measure may have reflected depressive symptoms at admission, but many schizophrenic patients with poor social and vocational skills, low self-esteem, and living in social isolation may be particularly defenseless when faced with adversity.

As adverse life events are known to be associated with the onset of depression (58, 59), these two studies support the notion that schizophrenic patients who experience adverse life events in the postdischarge period become demoralized and depressed and are then at increased risk to commit suicide. The reality of a schizophrenic patient again finding himself in difficulties within a few weeks or months of discharge may compound his feelings of hopelessness and helplessness and may mitigate against seeking either an earlier outpatient appointment or help from the emergency services. Anderson (81) described this well: "Since the schizophrenic individual has severe problems in coping with stress, it is during the posthospitalization period that suicidal risk is heightened. Confronted with the reality of returning to family and community life, the patient often feels his problems are impossible to resolve. His feelings of hopelessness about his situation may become overwhelming and lead to suicidal behavior."

Farberow and co-workers (51) noted that "the tranquilizing drugs, which reduced the disturbance, anxiety, and depression in the hospital did not necessarily provide the patient with better means to cope with the stresses of life away from the hospital" and that the suicide patients had needed to "develop new adaptive mechanisms for facing stressful life situations." They also noted that "It was only when passes or leaves were considered or given that there was a return of the anxiety and tension previously shown under stress." They suggested careful evaluation of both the supportiveness and stressfulness of the environment into which the patient is to be discharged, taking into account not only the reality of the situation but also the patient's feelings about it.

PREDICTION OF SUICIDE

In general the prediction of suicide is confounded by the prediction of too many "false positives" and "false negatives" (82, 83) (see discussion in Chapter 12). Shaffer and co-workers (49) tried to predict which schizophrenic patient would commit suicide. As the result of a 5-year follow-up study of 361 schizophrenic patients admitted to Johns Hopkins Hospital, 12 patients were known to have committed suicide. Their case folders were interspersed with those of a random sample of 75 patients known to be alive. Two research assistants scored each patient on two modified suicide risk scales, and two experienced psychiatrists "blindly" examined the folders and conjointly assessed on an 11-point clinical scale each patient's risk of eventual suicide. There were no significant differences between the two groups on any of 14 items on the two suicide risk scales, nor on their total scores. The suicides did have significantly higher mean scores on the clinical raters' suicide risk scale, and significantly more of them had made a previous suicide attempt. A multiple linear regression analysis revealed that four clinical items (the number of past attempts, alcohol abuse, sex, and age) made significant independent contributions to the clinical prediction, though together they failed to increase the prediction of suicide. The number of previous suicide attempts was found to be the most important single variable associated with suicide. However, the problem that prediction of an infrequent event like suicide predicts too many "false positives" was well illustrated, as 20.7% of the patients had high "suicidality" scores on the two raters' clinical scale but only 3.3% of the patients acutally committed suicide.

Studies have suggested that risk factors for suicide in schizophrenics include being young and male, having a relapsing illness, having been depressed in the past, being currently depressed, having been admitted in the last period of psychiatric contact with accompanying depressive symptoms or suicidal ideas, having recently changed from in- to outpatient care, and being socially isolated (84). Recently Drake and co-workers set out to determine which of these previously reported factors distinguished 15 schizophrenic patient suicides from 89 living schizophrenic patients. They, too, found that the suicides were young, the majority were male and had a chronic illness with numerous exacerbations and remissions (a mean 6.8 admissions during a mean 8.4 years of illness), significantly more of the suicides had made a past suicide threat (67%), and at their last hospitalization significantly more were depressed (80%), felt inadequate (80%), hopeless (60%), and had suicidal ideation (73%); 70% of the outpatient suicides killed themselves within 6 months of discharge, and significantly more of the suicides lived alone (60%).

These risk factors may well be useful in the acute short term suicide risk assessment of schizophrenic patients. However, as Shaffer and co-workers (49) showed, they are probably of limited value in the long range prediction of eventual suicide. Roy et al recently obtained follow-up information for 100 schizophrenic patients admitted a mean 4½ years earlier to the National Institute of Mental Health (85). Follow-up revealed that six patients had subsequently committed suicide. Using these risk factor items and combinations of items, they were able to identify only two of the six suicides while identifying many "false positives." Thus, at this time, the long range prediction of suicide in schizophrenic patients is not a practical proposition. However, research examining various long term interventions in schizophrenic patients who develop feelings of helplessness, hopelessness, and depression and who are considered to be at high risk for eventually committing suicide, may be useful.

Acknowledgment. Thanks are due to Andrea Hobbs for secretarial services.

References

1. Bleuler E: *Dementia Praecox or the Group of Schizophrenias.* New York, International Universities Press, 1950, 488.
2. Rennie T: Follow-up study of five hundred patients with schizophrenia admitted to the hospital from 1913 to 1923. *Arch Neurol Psychiatry* 41:877–891, 1939.
3. Markowe M, Steinert J, Heyworth-Davies F: Insulin and chlorpromazine in schizophrenia: a ten-year comparative study. *Br J Psychiatry* 113:1101–1106, 1967.
4. Winokur G, Tsuang M: The Iowa 500: suicide in mania, depression and schizophrenia. *Am J Psychiatry* 132:650–651, 1975.
5. McGlashan T: The Chestnut Lodge follow-up study. II. Long term outcome of schizophrenia and affective disorders. *Arch Gen Psychiatry* 41:586–601, 1984.
6. Miles P: Conditions predisposing to suicide: a review. *J Nerv Ment Dis* 164:231–246, 1977.
7. Pokorny A: Suicide rates in various psychiatric disorders. *J Nerv Ment Dis* 139:499–506, 1964.
8. Evenson R, Wood J, Nuttall E, Cho D: Suicide rates among public mental health patients. *Acta Psychiatr Scand* 66:254–264, 1982.
9. Wilkinson G: The suicide rate in schizophrenia. *Br J Psychiatry* 140:138–141, 1982.
10. Sleten I, Brown R, Evenson R, Altman H: Suicide in mental hospital patients. *Dis Nerv Syst* 33:328–335, 1972.
11. Flood R, Seager C: A retrospective examination of psychiatric case records of patients who subsequently committed suicide. *Br J Psychiatry* 114:443–450, 1968.
12. Roy A: Risk factors for suicide in psychiatric patients. *Arch Gen Psychiatry* 39:1089–1095, 1982.
13. Rorsman B: Suicide among Swedish psychiatric patients. *Soc Psychiatry* 8:140–144, 1978.
14. Dublin L: *Suicide. A Sociological and Statistical Study.* New York, Roland Press, 1963.
15. Barraclough B, Bunch J, Nelson B, Sainsbury P: A hundred cases of suicide. *Br J Psychiatry* 125:355–373, 1974.
16. Eastwood R, Peacocke J: Suicide, diagnosis and age. *Can Psychiatr Assoc J* 20:447–449, 1975.
17. Roy A: Suicide in chronic schizophrenia. *Br J Psychiatry* 141:171–177, 1982.
18. Hogan T, Awad G: Pharmacotherapy and suicide risk in schizophrenia. *Can J Psychiatry* 28:277–281, 1983.
19. Breier A, Astrachan B: Characterization of schizophrenic patients who commit suicide. *Am J Psychiatry* 141:206–209, 1984.
20. Drake R, Gates C, Cotton P, Whittaker A: Suicide among schizophrenics. Who is at risk? *J Nerv Ment Dis* 172:613–617, 1984.
21. Wilkinson G, Bacon N: A clinical and epidemiological survey of parasuicide and suicide in Edinburgh schizophrenics. *Psychol Med* 14:899–912, 1984.
22. Langley G, Bayatti N: Suicide in Exe Vale Hospital, 1972–1981. *Br J Psychiatry* 145:463–467, 1984.
23. Virkkunen M: Suicide in schizophrenia and paranoid psychosis. *Acta Psychiatr Scand (Suppl)* 250:1–305, 1974.
24. Aziz A, Salama A, Sizemore D: Observations on suicide among hospitalized schizophrenic patients. *Hosp Community Psychiatry* 33:940–941, 1982.

25. Waltzer H: Suicide risk in young schizophrenics. *Gen Hosp Psychiatry* 6:219–225, 1984.
26. Tsuang M: Suicide in schizophrenics, manics, depressives and surgical controls: a comparison with general population suicide mortality. *Arch Gen Psychiatry* 35:153–155, 1978.
27. Haugland G, Craig T, Goodman A, Siegel C: Mortality in the era of deinstitutionalization. *Am J Psychiatry* 140:848–852, 1983.
28. Warnes H: Suicide in schizophrenia. *Dis Nerv Sys* 29:35–40, 1968.
29. Noreik K: Attempted suicide and suicide in functional psychoses. *Acta Psychiatr Scand* 52:81–106, 1975.
30. Robins E, Murphy G, Wilkinson R, et al: Some clinical observations in the prevention of suicide based on a study of 134 successful suicides. *Am J Public Health* 49:888–898, 1959.
31. Loranger A: Sex differences in age at onset of schizophrenia. *Arch Gen Psychiatry* 41:157–161, 1984.
32. Seeman M: Gender and the onset of schizophrenia: neurohumoral influences. *Psychiatr J Univ Ottawa* 6:136–138, 1981.
33. Levine R: Sex differences in schizophrenia: timing or subtypes. *Psychol Bull* 90:432–444, 1981.
34. Leventhal D, Schuck J, Rothstein H: Gender differences in schizophrenia. *J Nerv Ment Dis* 172:464–467, 1984.
35. Salokangas R: Prognostic implications of the sex of schizophrenic patients. *Br J Psychiatry* 142:145–151, 1983.
36. Cohen S, Leonard C, Farberow N, Shneidman E: Tranquilizers and suicide in the schizophrenic patient. *Arch Gen Psychiatry* 11:312–321, 1964.
37. Black D, Warrack G, Winokur G: The Iowa Record-Linkage Study. III. Excess mortality among patients with functional disorders. *Arch Gen Psychiatry* 42:82–88, 1984.
38. Yarden P: Observations on suicide in chronic schizophrenics. *Compr Psychiatry* 15:325–333, 1974.
39. Copas J, Robin A: Suicide in psychiatric inpatients. *Br J Psychiatry* 141:503–511, 1982.
40. Watkins C, Gilbert J, Bass W: The persistent suicidal patient. *Am J Psychiatry* 125:1590–1593, 1969.
41. Niskanen P, Lonnqvist J, Achte K, Rinta-Mänty R: Suicides in Helsinki Psychiatric Hospitals in 1964–1972. *Psychiatr Fenn*, 275–280,1974.
42. Pokorny A, Kaplan H: Suicide following psychiatric hospitalization. *J Nerv Ment Dis* 162:119–125, 1976.
43. Stein G: Dangerous episodes occurring around the time of discharge of four chronic schizophrenics. *Br J Psychiatry* 141:586–589, 1982.
44. Roy A, Glaister G: Suicide in psychiatric patients. *Psychiatr J Univ Ottawa* 9:42–44, 1984.
45. Planasky K, Johnson R: The occurrence and characteristics of suicidal preoccupations and acts in schizophrenia. *Acta Psychiatr Scand* 47:473–483, 1971.
46. Roy A, Mazonson A, Pickar D: Attempted suicide in chronic schizophrenia. *Br J Psychiatry* 144:303–306, 1984.
47. Sainsbury P: Clinical aspects of suicide and its prevention. *Br J Hosp Med* 19:156–164, 1978.
48. Roy A: Suicide and psychiatric patients. *Psychiatr Clin North Am* 8:227–241, 1985.
49. Shaffer J, Perlin S, Schmidt C, Stephens S: The prediction of suicide in schizophrenia. *J Nerv Ment Dis* 159:349–355, 1974.
50. Dingman C, McGlashan T: Discriminating characteristics of suicide: Chestnut Lodge follow-up sample including patients with affective disorder, schizophrenia and schizoaffective disorder. *J Nerv Ment Dis*, in press.
51. Fareberow N, Shneidman E, Leonard C: Suicide among schizophrenic mental hospital patients. In Fareberow N, Shneidman S (eds): *The Cry for Help*. New York, McGraw-Hill, 1961, chap 6.
52. Levy S, Southcombe R: Suicide in a state hospital for the mentally ill. *J Nerv Ment Dis* 117:504–514, 1953.
53. Beisser A, Blanchette J: A study of suicides in a mental hospital. *J Dis Nerv Syst* 22:365–369, 1961.

112 / *Suicide*

54. Bolin R, Wright R, Wilkinson M, Lindner C: Survey of suicide among patients on home leave from a mental hospital. *Psychiatr Q* 42:81–89, 1968.
55. Fernando S, Storm V: Suicide among psychiatric patients of a district general hospital. *Psychol Med* 14:661–672, 1984.
56. Bunch J: Recent bereavement in relation to suicide. *J Psychosom Res* 16:361–366, 1972.
57. Paykel E, Prusoff B, Myers J: Suicide attempts and recent life events. *Arch Gen Psychiatry* 32:327–333, 1975.
58. Paykel E, Myers J, Dienelt M, Klerman G, Lindenthal J, Pepper M: Life events and depression. *Arch Gen Psychiatry* 21:753–760, 1969.
59. Roy A, Thompson R, Kennedy S: Depression in chronic schizophrenia. *Br J Psychiatry* 142:465–470, 1983.
60. Knesevich J, Zalcman S, Clayton P: Six year follow-up of patients with carefully diagnosed good and poor prognosis schizophrenia. *Am J Psychiatry* 140:1507–1509, 1983.
61. Caton C, Goldstein J, Serrano O: The impact of discharge planning on chronic schizophrenic patients. *Hosp Community Psychiatry* 35:255–262, 1984.
62. Johnstone E, Owens D, Gold A, Crow T, Macmillan F: Schizophrenic patients discharged from hospital—a follow-up study. *Br J Psychiatry* 145:586–590, 1984.
63. McCreadie R, Robinson A, Wilson O: The Scottish survey of chronic day patients. *Br J Psychiatry* 145:626–630, 1984.
64. DeAlarcon R, Carney M: Severe depressive mood changes following slow release intramuscular fluphenazine injection. *Br J Psychiatry* 3:564–567, 1969.
65. Roy A: Depression in chronic paranoid schizophrenia. *Br J Psychiatry* 137:138–139, 1980.
66. Roy A: Depression in the course of chronic undifferentiated schizophrenia. *Arch Gen Psychiatry* 38:296–300, 1981.
67. Johnson D: Studies of depressive symptoms in schizophrenia. *Br J Psychiatry* 139:89–101, 1981.
68. Roy A: Do neuroleptics cause depression. *Biol Psychiatry* 19:771–781, 1984.
69. Shear M, Frances A, Weiden P: Suicide associated with akathisia and depot fluphenazine treatment. *J Clin Psychopharmacol* 3:235–236, 1983.
70. Lehmann HE, Cancro R: Schizophrenia: clinical features. In Kaplan HI, Sadock BJ (eds): *Comprehensive Textbook of Psychiatry*, ed 4. Baltimore, Williams & Wilkins, 1984, vol 1.
71. Lehmann H, Ban T: Nature and frequency of the suicide syndrome, twenty years ago and today in the English-speaking community of the Province of Quebec. *Laval Med* 38:93–95, 1967.
72. Kraepelin E: *Dementia Praecox and Paraphrenia*. New York, Krieger, 1971.
73. Roy A: Suicide: a multidetermined act. *Psychiatr Clin North Am* 8:243–250, 1985.
74. Garralda E: Psychotic children with hallucinations. *Br J Psychiatry* 145:74–77, 1984.
75. Breier A, Strauss J: The role of social relationships in the recovery from psychotic disorders. *Am J Psychiatry* 141:949–955, 1984.
76. Wilson G: Suicide in psychiatric patients who have received hospital treatment. *Am J Psychiatry* 125:64–69, 1968.
77. Virkkunen M: Attitude to psychiatric treatment before suicide in schizophrenia and paranoid psychosis. *Br J Psychiatry* 128:47–49, 1976.
78. Baechler J: *Suicide*. New York, Basic Books, 1979, p 229.
79. Temoche A, Pugh T, MacMahon B: Suicide rates amongst current and former mental institution patients. *J Nerv Ment Dis* 138:124–130, 1964.
80. Winokur G: Quoted in *Clinical Psychiatry News*, February, 1984, p 34.
81. Anderson N: Suicide in schizophrenia. *Perspect Psychiatr Care* 11: 106–112, 1973.
82. Pokorny A: Prediction of suicide in psychiatric patients. *Arch Gen Psychiatry* 40:249–257, 1983.
83. Murphy G: On suicide prediction and prevention. *Arch Gen Psychiatry* 40:343–344, 1983.
84. Drake R, Gates C, Whitaker A, Cotton P: Suicide among schizophrenics: a review. *Compr Psychiatry* 26:90–100, 1985.
85. Roy A, Schreiber J, Mazonson A, Pickar D: Suicidal behavior in chronic schizophrenia: a follow-up study. *Can J Psychiatry*, in press.

8

Suicide in Neurosis and Personality Disorder

C. P. Seager, M.D., F.R.C.Psych.

Conventional wisdom has it that suicide is a common occurrence in psychotic conditions, particularly affective disorders and schizophrenia. A number of studies reviewing coroners' reports estimate that 30 to 89% of suicide victims demonstrate evidence of formal depressive illness at the time of death (1). Taking into account the fact that coroners' inquests produce a legal opinion based on circumstantial evidence rather than a medical opinion, one can conclude with Holding and Barraclough (2) that there is a high psychiatric morbidity both in past medical history and just before death. Since the principal witness is not available to provide an authoritative statement, conclusions must be at best problematical, but by their very consistency suggest a common thread running through the immediate presuicide emotional and cognitive functioning of the person concerned.

A diagnosis of depressive disorder in such circumstances begs even more questions than that wizened old stager, the issue of diagnosis in psychiatry. It can almost be taken for granted that someone who commits felo de se must feel at the end of their resources, that life has nothing further to offer, and that all is hopeless and black. It is therefore hardly surprising that suicide notes, whether dealing with the emotional state of the individual or setting out a last will and testament, including the venting of anger and aggression against those left behind, should still be construed as demonstrating an affective disorder of severe degree. After all, compulsory detention in hospital is usually initiated on the basis that the individual is behaving in such a way as to endanger the health of that individual or others.

One can look to the literature and find some interesting and useful views suggesting that psychiatric disorders in general, and neurotic and personality disorders in particular, have a specific mortality in which suicide plays an important part. Halbwachs' (3) *The Causes of Suicide* quotes Durkheim, who devoted the first chapter of his book to the study of suicide and psychopathic states. He could have found an indication of the physical and mental states of the suicide in the very numerous statistics on motives which most countries publish. However, he categorically refuses to resort to such data:

> "What are called statistics of the motives of suicide," (Durkheim wrote) "are actually statistics of the opinions concerning such motives of officials, often of lower officials, in charge of this information services .... We make it a rule not to employ in our studies such uncertain and uninstructive data."

Halbwachs comments at length on the psychiatric causes of suicide, and although he uses the term "psychopathic" in the sense that we would use "affective," he also comments on a number of patients with "deep-seated anxiety" (no sign of imbalance) as well as suicides of drunkards in his total. It is not clear from his table how many of these were actual suicides since he includes both suicides and attempts. He goes on to challenge the widely held view that "suicides, all suicides almost without exception," are explained by "the fit of anguish produced during the period of depression in recurrent manic depressive psychosis amongst subjects who have an emotional temperament." He recognizes that there could well be two clearly distinct categories of suicide. Perhaps 20 or 30% have psychopathic causes, i.e., psychosis, usually manic-depressive, but in the remainder one must look for a psychophysiological thesis. He assumes that at the moment in any individual who commits suicide, and perhaps for some hours or even days preceding, there would be some trouble of the nervous and cerebral functions, more or less deep seated, but always real. From this must result a psychic state similar to those found in the neuroses, of anguish, depression, etc.

However Halbwachs distinguishes between psychopathic suicides—those occurring in the midst of affective disorders—and normal suicides in response to personal and social events, recognizing that sociological factors play a major part in both. The mental disorder isolates the individual from the environment just as much as the normal person is isolated by bereavement, by convictions in the court, and by physical disability. He chides those psychiatrists who go too far when they conclude that social influence have no effect at all on individuals suffering from mental disorder. These comments, published in Paris in 1930, have continuing relevance in the 1980s when many more individuals seek and expect treatment in the community rather than isolated from their fellows by the walls of a mental institution.

Pokorny (4), in a widely quoted study of former patients of a Texas Veterans Administration hospital followed up over a 15-year period, calculated the suicide rates on the basis of 100,000 patients/year. He estimated that depression accounted for 566, schizophrenia for 167, neurosis for 119, personality disorder for 130, alcoholism for 133, and organic brain syndrome for 78. Thus individuals diagnosed as suffering from neurosis and personality disorder accounted for a quarter of the suicide rate. Babigian and Odoroff (5) examined a wider group of inpatients and outpatients undergoing various forms of psychiatric treatment. They found a risk of death 2½ to 3 times higher than the general population with a suicide rate of between 8 and 11/100,000. Kerr et al (6), in a study of 135 patients with various affective disorders followed up for a 2-year period, found two men with a diagnosis of anxiety state and one with depression who had committed suicide. Greer and Cawley (7) noted a 2.8% suicide rate in the 5-year follow-up of neurotic patients.

Sims (8), among others, has highlighted the increased mortality in patients suffering from various forms of neurosis. In a study of 166 patients treated in 1959 and followed up for 10 years, there were 20 deaths with 3 of these due to suicide and 5 ascribed to probable or quasisuicide, although not so identified by the coroner. A further 12 died of natural causes. Sims and Prior (9) repeated the study on a larger group of patients, finding 139 deaths amongst 1482 patients. Suicides and accidents contributed disproportionately, especially during the earlier follow-up period, but there was still a markedly increased mortality from combined categories of nervous, respiratory, and cardiovascular disease. Those who died (10) were suffering from more severe psychiatric conditions, as measured by specific criteria. Sims (11), summarizing his work in this field, drew attention to the relatively high incidence of suicide deaths in the first 2 years of follow-up compared with the more even death rate due to other causes. He emphasized the need for continuing arrangements to follow up patients for a longer period after discharge from hospital to try to reduce their risk of early demise.

Roy (12), comparing 90 psychiatric patients who committed suicide with matched controls, demonstrated high levels of factors which would normally be considered representative of personality disorders and nonspecific depressive disorders. Evidence suggests that individuals with neurotic problems and personality disorders form a more vulnerable group of individuals, susceptible to both physical disorders and suicidal behavior; both contribute to a higher mortality rate than expected in the general population. This does not take into account the more chronic forms of suicide, such as smoking, overeating, alcohol, and drug dependency, which are less likely to be picked up in such surveys.

This issue of a differential response to stress is of particular significance at a time when major economic factors produce unemployment, malnutrition, anomie, social isolation, despair, and apathy. Platt (13) has reviewed the extensive literature on unemployment and suicidal behavior. He concluded that there was firm evidence of an association between the two but that the nature of this association remained highly problematic. It is interesting to speculate about the role of welfare benefits in cushioning the unemployed from the full effects of economic disaster, compared with the apathy and despair engendered by a total separation from prospects of participating in the still current Protestant work ethic.

CONSEQUENCES OF SUICIDE

The typical coroner's verdict used to state: "lost his life whilst the balance of his mind was disturbed." This provided a veneer of respectable excuse to justify an antireligious and antisocial mode of behavior. It also had legal connotations in the days when suicide was a crime, since the benefits of such a felony could be withheld from the family. This was relevant in terms of a will and of insurance policies.

Modern verdicts are more blunt, stating simply: "Suicide" or "He took his own life." Social pressures still ensure that the coroner gives his verdict only when the available evidence fully justifies the conclusion, not on a balance of probabilities but without reasonable doubt. In England, Lord Widgery (14) the Lord Chief Justice, warned coroners when returning a case to the court after appeal by disquieted relatives that "I must impress on Coroners that an open verdict is no reflection on them. It does not mean that they are not doing their job properly. There are many cases where an open verdict is right . . . . The Coroner's approach seems to have ignored one of the most important rules—that suicide must not be presumed because it is the most likely explanation. If it cannot be proved by the evidence, he should find an open verdict."

People take a long time to change and a verdict of suicide is still a slur on the family and friends and also on the professionals who made a "mistake" and allowed someone to slip through their fingers. Individuals with psychotic conditions who commit suicide are usually seen as excusing those around them from some degree of blame. It is seen more as a response to illness in the way that death from cancer can be looked upon as part of the natural process.

Where the diagnosis is one of neurotic or personality disorder the family become angry, partly because of a background of guilt and rejection as the patient has gone through many sessions of complaint, recrimination, suicidal threats, and manipulated behavior. Professional staff also become angry and attempt to rationalize their rejection of the patient. "He is quite sane—he knows what he is doing and must take the consequences of his own actions. Every time we rescue him we are reinforcing his attention-seeking behavior."

It would be more appropriate to recognize that attention-seeking behavior should be equated with attention-needing behavior. The issue is how best to respond in a constructive way. The role of the professional helper is to recognize the need of the patient to form a therapeutic relationship which allows a recognition and identification of those activities which are maladaptive, to modify them in a constructive manner, and to help the patient find a more appropriate pattern of behavior.

In the meantime, suicidal activity remains a risk for the patient who does not conform and for the professional staff who become irritated by his apparent inability to accept help which is offered. Flood and Seager (15), in a retrospective study of patients who had committed suicide, found no obvious factors distinguishing those who had died from a comparison group, apart from a tendency to be labeled as uncooperative or attention-seeking or to have taken their own discharge from hospital against medical advice. Farberow and his colleagues (16) noted a similar finding labeling their patients "dependent-dissatisfied," making repetitive demands on others regardless of effect and thus alienating them. More recently Morgan (17) in his book *Death Wishes?* described the case histories of 8 inpatient suicides who were so provocative, difficult, and unreasonable that the staff ultimately felt hostile toward them before their suicides. He developed this further in a recent symposium (18) in which he dealt with the total of 26 patients of whom 12 were previously reported and 14 further patients with diagnoses varying from depressive illness, 9; obsessional compulsive neurosis, 1; chronic schizophrenia, 1; anorexia nervosa and bulimia, 1; and personality disorder, 2. He recognized the process of "terminal or malignant alienation" which may be provoked by a recurrent relapse or difficult behavior. This may be common in the week or days before suicide occurs. In the final act of suicide the attitudes of others and the life difficulties may be just as important as the psychopathology of the person who killed himself.

In the same symposium Crammer postulates two hypotheses, both of which are capable of testing. One possibility is that an antisuicidal ward is one with a calm routine carried out by staff who are themselves unworried and confident of the immediate future. Inpatient suicides would then occur predominantly when this calm is broken for any reason, when routine is disrupted and the staff is disturbed. The second hypothesis emphasizes the importance of interpersonal relationships and predicts that suicide may occur where there is a failure to make any relationship with a staff member or fellow patient. These hypotheses are not mutually exclusive.

The family of a suicide may have been as much in need of attention prior to the act as the victim. After the act the victim is beyond help but the family remains (19). In addition to the issues which were relevant in the life of the suicide, factors of guilt and recrimination add to the normal processes of grieving. Such individuals feel particularly isolated and neglected. This may perhaps be because they are indeed neglected or because their own anxieties and guilt deprive them of the opportunities of seeking help from friends or professional supporters. One frequently reads reports of suicide studies where the family were not interviewed as it was thought that this would be too traumatic for them. This delicacy may be based on legitimate empathic consideration but may also be a rationalization protecting the investigtors from an embarrassing and uncomfortable outpouring of necessary emotional abreaction. A few relatives of patients who have committed suicide while under treatment have commented afterward how lost they felt because no one was prepared to offer help, support, advice, or even information about what had gone wrong. One cannot know about the many who had no contact with the psychiatric services.

MULTIPLE SUICIDES

If one looks at the response to the death of an individual by the "significant others," the near relatives and close friends, one can conceive of a continuum of emotional reaction and consequent behavior. Where death is from natural causes, particularly when it is predicted, there may be feelings of grieving and loss modified by a sense of relief that the waiting is over and possibly a release from pain and distress, both for the dead individual and for the survivors. Where death is sudden, unexpected, or takes place in an individual before the normal and expected time span, emotional reactions tend to be more intense and behavior may be exaggerated. Still stronger are the emotional and behavior responses caused by death at the hand of another, whether it be murder, accident, or negligence. There appears to be a pattern of increasing emotionality and behavioral response depending on the degree of unexpectedness and culpability surrounding the death.

It is recognized that there is an increased mortality amongst widows and widowers during the year following their bereavement (20). A more extreme variant on this situation is where the spouse or other close associate of the dead person recognizes that the loss is too great to tolerate and decides to join the departed person in death. This may in itself result in suicide at some point following the death of the first individual.

Rarely, according to psychiatrists, but more more commonly if one reads the newspapers, one sees reports of suicide pacts where two individuals agree that life without each other would be impossible and separately but together decide to take their own lives. Such situations invariably attract newpaper comments; reference to the index of the *London Times* newspaper shows examples of many such events with spouses, mothers or fathers and children, lovers either heterosexual or homosexual, and siblings participating in a joint action of self-destruction. It is difficult to know the true rate of such actions because national newspapers in Great Britain cater to a population of perhaps 50 million and draw their information from this wide field as well as occasional reports from abroad.

Psychiatrists, on the other hand, usually limit their surveys to relatively small populations and may concentrate on one or other aspect of a complex series of patterns. Cohen (21) studied 68 pacts over a 3-year period. These formed 1 in 300 suicides of that period. The vast majority, 72%, were pacts between spouses, while only 5 were between unhappy lovers. Hemphill and Thornley (22) commented on the rarity of reports and the fact that survivors of pacts are unusual, as also did Cohen. They referred to the lack of formal psychotic illness but the presence of an intense and exclusive relationship resulting in "an encapsulated unit" within which the couple interact. West (23) discussed a special case of multiple deaths where murder is followed by suicide. In this case a high proportion of the deaths take place in the context of a depressive illness on the part of the initiator of the act who destroys one or more close associates, usually members of the family, as a result of depressive ideas and then commits suicide. Ohara (24) commented particularly on the frequency of mother/child suicides in Japan where the mother forces the child to take poison and then does the same thing herself. This was similarly described in *Keesing's Contemporary Archives* (25) where there was mass suicide of followers of the United States Peoples' Temple Sect under the leadership of the Reverend James Jones. Mothers were encouraged to kill their children by administering orange juice poisoned with cyanide before killing themselves.

Parry-Jones (26) discussed the legal aspect of suicide pacts and the finding amongst 80 cases reported to the director of public prosecution that incomplete pacts were twice as numerous as completed ones. This is in contradistinction to the findings of both Cohen and Hemphill and Thornley.

In a more recent review of suicide pacts, Rosen (27) concluded that approximately 1% of all suicides are suicide pacts in the U.K. and Western Europe, and found some suggestion that they may form over 3% of suicides in Japan. There is obviously a strong relationship between suicides and folie a deux, although the presence of delusional ideas is unusual in the information available about suicide pacts. Nevertheless, there is a stong interdependence between the couple forming an encapsulated unit which illness or other unexpected circumstances threatens to destroy. Christodoulou (28) and Salih (29) both described suicide pacts in relationship to folie a deux. Rosenbaum (30) suggests that it is likely that the instigator, usually male and psychiatrically ill, will die while the cooperator, female and not psychiatrically ill, will survive. This view is not held by all writers on this subject, although it is in keeping with the report by Christodoulou. Fishbain and colleagues (31) carried out a controlled study of suicide pacts. They identified 20 such pacts and compared these with 120 randomly selected single suicides from the same time area. This study tended to confirm previous findings. For example, 70% of the pacts were between spouses, and only 20% were between lovers. There was overwhelming support for the relevance of social isolation. There was a high incidence of firearms as a means of suicide, although other aggressive and violent means of suicide were uncommon. When one considers the cultural connotations of suicidal behavior, it is remarkable that there is a high degree of concordance amongst reports from such disparate areas as England, Florida, and South Africa.

DRUG DEPENDENCY AND SUICIDE

The slow suicide of drug dependency is occasionally accelerated by a miscalculated excess of drug or a specific decision to bring to an end the pressures and chronic ill health of illegal drug taking. It is often difficult to determine the cause when a drug addict is found dead. There may be evidence of a high dose of the usual drug, but this may be taken with a view to suicide, as experimentation to achieve greater heights of release, or brought about by an accidental administration of a more pure and less contaminated version of the usual supply. At other times the situation is clearer since the death is related to some other form of destruction, such as jumping or hanging. Even then, the situation may not be clear since the fantasies induced by hallucinogenic drugs are said to produce beliefs of nonhumans powers or immortality which, when put to the test, prove unfounded.

Suicide due to opiate addiction and by the use of opiates is neither new nor rare. Clarke (32) describes techniques familiar to present-day drug users, including going to several pharmacists to accumulate doses of laudanum; the principle, if not the drug, is the same.

He describes a suicide pact with opium occurring in Chester in 1861 and again in Glasgow in 1899 and Liverpool in 1904. During the First World War interference with the manufacture of munitions due to excessive cocaine, opium, and alcohol in Britain resulted in the passing in 1916 of the Defence of the Realm Act (DORA), confirmed after the war by the Dangerous Drugs Act of 1920 making drugs containing more than 0.2% morphine or 0.1% heroin available only by prescription.

A number of follow-up studies of narcotic addicts have demonstrated a relatively high death rate. As already indicated, it is not always clear whether this is due to suicide or other factors. Vaillant (33) reported 16 deaths in a 12-year follow-up of 100 male narcotic addicts in New York. James (34) described 39 deaths, a rate of 2.7% with five suicides and four overdoses which were probable suicides. He also commented that imprisonment carries its own suicide risk of 3 to 5% with death occurring during the period of drug withdrawal. However, in a more extensive review of suicide in prison, Topp (35) found a suicide rate of 42/100,000 daily average population and 14 suicides/100,000 receptions into custody. One-third were on remand and two-thirds had been sentenced. In 82% there were indications that emotional relationships were unsatisfactory. Seventy-nine percent were single or separated, 54% had been living in lodgings alone or were vagrants, and 45% had no known contact with relatives or friends. It was interesting to note that 30% had a drinking problem and 11% had a drug problem prior to conviction.

Bewley and colleagues (36) found that 23% of deaths in a group of heroin-dependent individuals were due to suicide and an additional 29% were caused by narcotic overdose or sudden unexpected death. They estimated that there was a 20 times greater risk of death amongst addicts than would be expected for that age group. In a related study, Bewley and Ben-Aire (37) found that 13% of inpatients were dead on follow-up, 8% due to overdose with opiates or barbiturates. Noble and colleagues (38) studied a group of over 1000 adolescent girls admitted to a remand home in London. A quarter of these girls used drugs and at follow-up 10 were dead, two from hanging and seven from an overdose; one other died from infective hepatitis. Thorley and colleagues (39) followed up heroin addicts attending a drug clinic. They traced 128 after 6 years and 12 of these (9%) were dead. The cause was not stated. Feuerlein (40) found the suicide rates 22 times higher than in the general population amongst the group of addicts and alcoholics. Stimson and colleagues (41) reported a separate 7-year follow-up of heroin addicts and found that 12% had died. Suicidal behavior was reported in two cases, but in the others the verdict was addiction to drugs with no specific mention of suicide.

More general studies of psychiatric follow-up such as Black et al (42) demonstrate a significantly higher observed mortality than that expected in neuroses, personality disorders, alcohol and other drug abusers, while Martin et al (43) comment on the higher mortality amongst patients diagnosed as having secondary depression related to antisocial personality, drug addiction, etc. They comment on the less effective treatment of affective disorders secondary to personality disorder or substance abuse partly because of the difficulties in treating the underlying problem and also because of lack of compliance on the part of such individuals.

CONCLUSION

Studies of suicide occurring among patients diagnosed as having personality disorders, neurosis, secondary affective disorders, or drug dependency and also in those individuals directed into penal rather than health institutions all show a suicide rate up to 20-fold greater than the general population. One can speculate whether the suicide occurs in the setting of a depressive response to dismal life circumstances or is a consequence of the same vulnerable personality who exhibits neurotic symptoms, psychopathic behavior, or a substance abuse. Whatever the explanation, these individuals do not encourage compassion, warmth, tenderness, or concern on the part of those who come in contact with them, whether family, friends, colleagues, or mental health professionals. Yet it is the responsibility of the latter—those who are trained to understand that behavior may be inappropriate, irrational, aggressive, destructive, uncooperative, or rejecting—to offer a constructive and therapeutic support which will allow the damaged individual to make some progress towards a solution rather than dissolution.

References

1. Shaw SP, Sims ACP: A survey of unexpected deaths among psychiatric in-patients. *Br J Psychiatry* 145:473 476, 1984.

2. Holding TA, Barraclough BM: Psychiatric morbidity in a sample of a London Coroner's Open Verdicts. *Br J Psychiatry* 127:133–143, 1975.
3. Halbwachs M: *The Causes of Suicide.* London, Routledge & Kegan Paul, 1978.
4. Pokorny AD: Suicide rates in various psychiatric disorders. *J Nerv Ment Dis* 139:499–506, 1964.
5. Babigian HM, Odorff CL The mortality experiences of a population with psychiatric illness. *Am J Psychiatry* 126:470–480, 1969.
6. Kerr TA, Schapira K, Roth M: The relationship between premature death and affective disorders. *Br J Psychiatry* 115:1277–1282, 1969.
7. Greer S, Cawley RH: *Some Observations on the Natural History of Neurotic Illness.* Archdall Medical Monograph no. 3. Sydney, Australia Publ, Co, 1966.
8. Sims A: Mortality in neurosis. *Lancet* 2:1072–1076, 1973.
9. Sims ACP, Prior P: Pattern of mortality in severe neuroses. *Br J Psychiatry* 133:299–305, 1978.
10. Sims ACP, Rudge BJ: Discrimination between neurotics who die and neurotics who live. *Acta Psychiatr Scand* 59:317–325. 1979.
11. Sims A: *Neurosis in Society.* London, Macmillan, 1983.
12. Roy A: Risk factors for suicide in psychiatric patients. *Arch Gen Psychiatry* 39:1089–1095, 1982.
13. Platt S: Unemployment and suicidal behavior. A review of the literature. *Soc Sci Med* 19:93–115, 1984.
14. Widgery, Lord Justice: Law reports. *Times*, April 23 and July 2, 1975.
15. Flood RA, Seager CP: A retrospective examination of psychiatric case records of patients who subsequently committed suicide. *Br J Psychiatry* 114:443–450, 1968.
16. Farberow NL, Shneidman ES, Neuringer C: Case history and hospitalization factors in suicides of neuropsychiatric hospital patients. *J Nerv Ment Dis* 142:32–44, 1966.
17. Morgan HG: *Death Wishes? The Understanding and Management of Deliberate Self-Harm.* John Wiley & Sons, New York, 1979.
18. Crammer JL: Symposium on suicide in hospital. *Br J Psychiatry* 145:459–476, 1984.
19. Shneidman ES: An overview: personality motivation and behavior theories. In Hankoff LD, Eisidler B, (eds): *Suicice: Theory and Clinical Aspects.* Littleton, MA, PSG Publishing Co, 1979.
20. Parkes CM: Recent bereavement as a cause of mental illness. *Br J Psychiatry* 110:198–204, 1964.
21. Cohen J: A study of suicide pacts. *Medico-Legal* 29:144–151, 1961.
22. Hemphill RE, Thornley FI: Suicide pacts. *South Afr Med J* 43:1335–1338, 1969.
23. West DJ: *Murder Followed by Suicide.* Cambridge, Heinmann, 1965.
24. Ohara K: Characteristics of suicide in Japan, especially of parent-child double suicide. *Am J Psychiatry* 120:382–385, 1963.
25. Mass suicide of followers of United States "People's Temple" sect. In *Keesing's Contemporary Archives*, 1979.
26. Parry-Jones W: Criminal law and complicity in suicide and attempted suicide. *Med Sci Law* 13:110–119, 1973.
27. Rosen BK: Suicide pacts: a review. *Psychol Med* 11:525–533, 1981.
28. Christodoulou GN: Two cases of folie a deux in husband and wife. *Acta Psychiatr Scand* 46:413–419, 1970.
29. Salih MA: Suicide pact in a setting of folie a deux. *Br J Psychiatry* 139:62–67, 1981.
30. Rosenbaum M: Crime and punishment. The suicide pact. *Arch Gen Psychiatry* 40:979–982, 1983.
31. Fishbain DA, D'achille L, Barsky S, Aldrich TE: A controlled study of suicide pacts. *J Clin Psychiatry* 45:154–157, 1984.
32. Clarke M: Suicides by opium and its derivatives in England and Wales 1850–1950. *Psychol Med* 2:237–242, 1985.
33. Vaillant GE: A twelve year follow up of New York narcotic addicts. 1. The relation of treatment to outcome. *Am J Psychiatry* 122:727–737, 1966.

34. James IP: Suicide and mortality amongst heroin addicts in Britain. *Br J Addict* 62:391–398, 1967.
35. Topp DO: Suicide in prison. *Br J Psychiatry* 134:24–27, 1979.
36. Bewley TH, Ben-Arie O, Pierce JI: Morbidity and mortality from heroin dependence. 1. Survey of heroin addicts known to Home Office. *Br Med J* 1:725–726, 1968.
37. Bewley TH, Ben-Arie O: Morbidity and mortality from heroin dependence. 2. Study of 100 consecutive in-patients. *Br Med J* 1:727–730, 1968.
38. Noble P, Hart T, Nation R: Correlates and outcome of illicit drug use by adolescent girls. *Br J Psychiatry* 120:497–504, 1972.
39. Thorley A, Oppenheime RE, Stimson GV: Clinic attendance and opiate prescription status of heroin addicts over a six year period. *Br J Psychiatry* 130:565–569, 1977.
40. Feuerlein W: Addiction and suicide. *Psychiatr Fenn Suppl*, 101–104, 1978.
41. Stimson GV, Oppenheimer E, Thorley A: Seven year follow-up of heroin addicts: drug use and outcome. *Br Med J* 1:1190–1192, 1979.
42. Black DW, Warrack G, Winokur G: The Iowa record-linkage study. 1. Suicides and accidental deaths among psychiatric patients. *Arch Gen Psychiatry* 42:71–75, 1985.
43. Martin RL, Cloninger R, Guze SB, Clayton PJ: Mortality in a follow-up of 500 psychiatric outpatients. 2. Cause-specific mortality. *Arch Gen Psychiatry* 42:58–66, 1985.

9

Completed Suicide

Eli Robins, M.D.

An old question that has been addressed by investigators concerns the difference in the planning of outcome by those who attempt and those who complete suicide. In the 1930s, von Andics (1), a Viennese psychiatrist, drew attention to the possibility that attempted suicide and completed suicide represent different phenomena, and, following her lead, other psychiatrists later pointed out that not only are attempted suicide and completed suicide different events, they occur in overlapping but different populations. Ettlinger's 1964 review (2) of 11 studies of attempted suicide indicated that, annually, from 1 to 2% of persons attempting suicide will eventually complete suicide. These studies, with widely varying follow-up periods as well as numbers of patients involved, uncovered a strikingly narrow incidence of subsequent completed suicide.

This chapter concerns itself with the subject of completed suicide and so it seems reasonable to try first to put into perspective the kinship (or relative lack thereof) of attempted and completed suicide. Many more people—5 to 10 times as many—attempt suicide than complete it. Thus, attempted suicide is much more obviously a symptom of other problems than it is a precursor or predictor of eventual completed suicide. Attempted suicide is associated far more often with hysteria, antisocial personality, and various paraphilias than it is with completed suicide. By the same token, hysteria, antisocial personality, and the various paraphilias are illnesses that rarely involve completed suicide as an outcome. Rather, the psychiatric illnesses that most frequently lead to completed suicide have been shown to be affective disorder, depressed phase, and alcoholism. Thus, while attempted suicide is certainly an important psychiatric phenomenon, its importance relative to completed suicide is a lot less than one might assume.

PSYCHIATRIC ILLNESS AND COMPLETED SUICIDE

Since the psychiatrist's most immediate aim in dealing with the question of suicide is to gain as much information as possible to enable himself/herself to recognize its risk in individual patients, perhaps the most direct approach is a review of clinical studies. There have been, to date, three studies in English involving 100 or more consecutive suicides (3–5). Thus, in three studies, undertaken over a 10-year period, one sees that, in combination, affective disorder, depressed phase (or depressive illness, as it is called by two of the groups) and alcoholism were found to be the diagnoses predominantly associated with completed suicide (70%—239 of the 342 suicides studied) (see Tables 9.1–9.3). At the same time, schizophrenia, which has had the

Table 9.1. Diagnostic Breakdown in 100 Cases of Suicide Studied in England (3)

Depressive illness	70%
Alcoholism	15%
Schizophrenia	3%
Phobic-anxiety state	3%
Barbiturate dependence	1%
Acute schizoaffective disorder	1%
Not mentally ill	7%

(Depressive illness + alcoholism = 85%)

Table 9.2. Diagnostic Breakdown in 108 Cases of Suicide Studied in Washington State (4)

Depressive illness	28%
Alcoholism	26%
Schizophrenia	11%
Personality and sociopathic disorders	9%
Organic brain syndrome	4%
Miscellaneous	3%
Unspecified psychiatric illness	15%
No psychological information	5%

(Depressive illness + alcoholism = 54%)

Table 9.3. Diagnostic Breakdown of 134 Suicides Studied in St. Louis (5)

Affective disorder, depressed phase	47%
Alcoholism	25%
Organic brain syndrome	4%
Schizophrenia	2%
Drug dependence	1%
Undiagnosed psychiatric illness	15%
Terminal medical illness	4%
Well	2%

(Affective disorder, depressed phase + alcoholism = 72%)

reputation of close association with suicide, was found to exist in a mean of only 5% of the overall samples and hysteria in less than 1%.

In two of these studies, 15% of each sample was found to fall into the "undiagnosed (or "unspecified") psychiatric illness" category. The St. Louis investigators separated their 20 undiagnosed subjects into subcategories called the "most like" groups—i.e., there were 11 subjects who, though undiagnosed, were "most like" sufferers from affective disorder, three who were "most like" alcoholics, and six whose symptoms seemed to fit most closely with one or another of the criteria for diagnoses in the miscellaneous group. (This miscellaneous group includes organic brain syndrome, schizophrenia, drug dependence, terminally medically ill, and well). Once one considers an undiagnosed group from this vantage point (albeit an educated hypothesis), it follows that the numbers of subjects from each "most like" category might be added to those in the definite diagnostic groups and the resulting figures add weight—an additional 10%—to the finding of the high rate of affective disorder and alcoholism among those who complete suicide (82% of the total St. Louis sample).

Affective Disorder and Suicide

It has been a problem for the psychiatry community to settle firmly on a good descriptive term for the disease now fairly commonly known as affective disorder. One reason for the difficulty is the disagreement about whether psychiatrists are dealing with one disease or more than one. To further complicate things, if we are dealing with only one, the implication must be that its various symptoms are examples of heterogeneous manifestations of a single underlying illness.

In the St. Louis study, it was found that all those subjects with affective disorder were in the depressed phase at the time of their deaths. Indeed, as far as could be determined, none of the 63 subjects with affective disorder had ever had a manic episode. This is an unusual finding. Most studies which describe depression and mania separately indicate a ratio of depression to mania of around 6:1. Barraclough et al (3), in fact, cite 11 (17%) of their 64 depressive suicides as having had previous episodes of mania, though none of the subjects were manic at the time of death. Dorpat and Ripley (4) did not, in their study, describe any of their depressed subjects as having had manic episodes, nor did they, in fact, refer to mania at all.

The depressed phase of affective disorder is an illness that causes a plethora of symptoms and makes life miserable for those affected. Even when an attack of affective disorder is mild, it is still noticeably disabling and debilitating. The mildly depressed person suffers from feelings of poor self-image, inadequacy, and "the blues." The person is often concerned about having some serious medical illness and about dying. These thoughts are frequent, repetitive, and difficult to avoid for any significant period of time.

In the most depressed person, there is a crescendo effect during which the patient feels more and more worthless and less and less hopeful that the disease will ever recede. Along with this may come the problems of increased slowness and sluggishness of movement (though some patients experience the opposite—motor agitation) and of speech, sometimes to the point of muteness. Other frequent complaints are those of inability to think, to concentrate, to feel emotion, and feeling that the "head is empty." Delusions such as incurability, general self-blame, illness as a punishment for sin, and abject poverty also occur. Hallucinations are encountered in about one-tenth of depressed subjects who are hospitalized for psychiatric reasons. An example is a criticizing voice accusing a patient of being the cause of his own problems.

The patient with an affective disorder is also virtually always afflicted with bodily symptoms. The lack of uninterrupted sleep, the presence of nausea, the loss of appetite, the resultant loss of weight, unrelieved pains, and trouble breathing combine to make life extremely unpleasant. There is also a deep sense of joylessness which involves a loss of interest in those aspects of life which are commonly associated with happiness—work, home, grandchildren, holidays, sex, reading, movies, company, etc.

Life becomes, for the depressed person, a painful existence without promise or expectation of relief. In the light of the description of such an existence, the reader may better understand the allure of suicide.

Alcoholism and Suicide

The three major studies of completed suicide referred to above show an average of 22% of all subjects diagnosed as having had alcoholism. The symptom which is common to virtually all alcoholics is weekly to daily drinking (94% drink daily). Many kinds of physical problems are related to daily drinking, but it is probable that the most widely destructive of the effects of alcoholism are not those upon the alcoholic subject's physical being, but those upon his and his loved ones' emotions. Typical of alcoholism, which is a long term illness, are frequent disruptions of subjects' affectional relationships. An alcoholic of long standing seems to undergo an almost unlimited number of troubles in his home life and still maintain the urge to renew relationships or form new ones after the most severe emotional upheavals. However, in suicides of alcoholics, it is most often the case that the suicidal act closely follows one last incident in a string of violated and re-created relationships. It seem that it is a matter, in alcoholism and suicide, of there being a straw that breaks the camel's back. What is not clear is why the individual camel's back breaks under the weight of a given straw at a given time. Because this question is of continuing interest to psychiatrists, an effort to answer it has been an aspect in studies of attempted suicide. In one such study (6), the question, "What was the chief reason for your attempt?" was included in interviews with such subjects. Persons suffering from affective disorder, depressed phase, most often gave personal reasons such as feelings of guilt or of hopelessness, while, in contrast, subjects suffering from alcoholism gave social reasons, such as family trouble, legal trouble, or loss of job.

Relatives of people who complete suicide provide numerous examples of the particular kinds of suffering experienced by and inflicted on others by alcoholic subjects. These include outbursts of anger causing danger to those close to the subject, disturbing the privacy and peace of strangers as well as of acquaintances and neighbors, living in isolation, violation of marriage to the point of separations and divorce, disregard for the welfare and emotional security of offspring, trouble with police as a result of drunk driving, automobile accidents, peace disturbance, fighting, and destruction of property, crass failure to provide financially and emotionally for those for whom the subject was legally responsible.

In addition to the social troubles and indignities inflicted by alcoholics on themselves and on others, there are the alcoholic-induced physical problems—cirrhosis, ascites, delirium tremens, alcoholic gastritis, anorexia, nausea, vomiting, and abdominal pain. Besides these frequent gastrointestinal symptoms, there are also many symptoms observed in the histories of the alcoholic subjects which are reminiscent of those seen in affective disorder, depressed phase. It can be assumed that in alcoholism these scattered symptoms similar to those of affective disorder may be manifestations of brain damage (due to head injuries). These symptoms are mainly those causing psychological pain, but also include a few, like outbursts of rage, which are potentially destructive to others. Some of those causing the alcoholic subjects psychological pain are suicidal ideas, disbelief in the possibility of recovery, sadness, prophecy of black future, and conviction of the loss of mind. Given the apparent difference in the pathogenesis of what sounds like the same symptoms, it is likely that they involve and affect differently diagnosed subjects in quite different ways.

The alcoholic is, of course, aware of society's expectation of "self-control," a possibility beyond the alcoholic's grasp. Thus, he is doubly afflicted and most likely to turn the blame on family, boss, friends—society as it accuses him. Years of alcoholism intensify the uselessness of this reasoning. The chronicity of alcoholism contrasts with the overwhelmingly episodic nature of affective disorder. In alcoholism, the disbelief in ever recovering has some basis in fact, and one can imagine a resultant feeling of hopelessness that would entertain suicide.

Other Illnesses and Suicide

Of the 342 subjects studied in the three major suicide investigations, 45 (13%) of them were diagnosed as suffering from psychiatric illnesses other than affective disorder and alcoholism: 18 were schizophrenics, 3 were drug addicts, 3 were suffering from a "phobic-anxiety state" (3), 9 had organic brain syndrome, 10 had "personality and sociopathic disorders" (4), and 1 suffered from acute "schizoaffective disorder" (3). As noted above, schizophrenia has been thought to be associated with a large proportion of deaths by suicide. That this is not the case has been shown in all three studies of 100 or more consecutive suicides and in a recent study of hospitalized psychiatric patients (7). In that study, by Shaffer et al, only 12 (3%) of 361 hospitalized patients diagnosed as having schizophrenia committed suicide within a 5-year observation period. The 10 subjects diagnosed as having had "personality and sociopathic disorders" were all from the group studied by Dorpat and Ripley, and it is difficult to know exactly what is meant by this particular combination of diagnostic terms. Two others of these miscellaneous psychiatric diagnoses did not always have counterparts in the three similar studies of suicide. While Barraclough et al found that 1% of their subjects were drug dependent, Dorpat and Ripley found none. And while Dorpat and Ripley's finding that 4% of their suicide subjects had had organic brain syndrome matched in the St. Louis finding, Barraclough et al made no diagnoses of organic brain syndrome. These matched and mismatched findings in the miscellaneous category suitably reflect the infrequency of suicide among people suffering from organic brain syndrome and drug dependence.

The prevalence of suicide among the terminally medically ill is proportionately far less than it is among people with organic brain syndrome or those with schizophrenia and less even than among those with drug dependence (3). And while suicide in organic brain syndrome, schizophrenia, and drug dependence is rare when compared with suicide in affective disorder, depressed phase, and in alcoholism, it is even rarer among people with terminal medical illness. Despite the devastation of fatal illnesses, suicide is so rarely associated with them that physicians do not usually consider it as a possible outcome.

SUICIDE AMONG THE "WELL"

Three of the suicide subjects in the St. Louis sample were diagnosed as "well." The reader may wonder—as indeed the investigators did—about these three who had neither terminal medical illness nor, as far as could be determined, psychiatric illness. In all three cases, the informants were candid about the subjects, but application of two sets of diagnostic criteria turned up no evidence of psychiatric illness. Thus the diagnosis, "undiagnosed psychiatric illness," did not apply. While there was evidence of physical illness in at least one of the three, the illness was not even potentially fatal. Neither of the two other subjects had, at the times of their suicides, any physical illnesses. The reader might ask an obvious question: "Since these three persons did actually take their own lives, were they not, by definition, depressed?" The answer must necessarily be that the suicidal act was the only overt, reported act interpretable as depressed, psychotic, drug induced, or psychiatrically abnormal. One such act is not enough on which to base a diagnosis. These cases, enigmatic as they are, are not unique to the St. Louis sample. Barraclough and his group of investigators considered seven subjects from their sample "not to be mentally ill." And Dorpat and Ripley's six subjects who were excluded from their sample because of the "unavailability of psychological information" probably fall into the same category, although this is not specifically stated in their report.

Suicide among the "well" is indeed mystifying, but the author believes that these seemingly "well" suicide subjects probably did suffer from psychiatric illness of one sort or another that simply did not manifest typically.

PREDICTORS OF SUICIDE

Obviously, there is no pathognomonic predictor of completed suicide. There are, however, a number of predictors that correlate with completed suicide and are helpful in predicting suicide. The continuing study of suicide shows that some predictors are better than others.

Age, sex, race, and psychiatric diagnosis in certain combinations are probably the most consistently accurate predictors of suicide and, by the same token, are in other combinations accurate in predicting a low risk of suicide. Completed suicide is more than 3 times as frequent in men as it is in women. The number of suicides by white men in the United States is 20 times the number of suicides by black men. The population ratio of whites to blacks is about 10:1. Therefore, the real ratio is approximately 2:1, white suicides to black suicides. The most complete record of suicide death *rates* for white men and black men, by age and color, is presented in the form of a cohort analysis covering 5-year intervals from 1952 to 1967 (8). Death rates for the cohorts were assessed every 5 years and there was an overall, slight, and insignificant upward trend in the suicide rate for blacks as compared with whites. The rate of suicide among white men over the age of 32 continues to increase with age and does so beyond age 80. The rate among black men, in contrast, rises more or less parallel with the white male rate to age 32, at which point the rates deviate markedly, the black rate remaining more or less steady from 32 to 80 as the white rate continues to rise. This deviation between black and white male suicide rates eventuates in an about 5:1 (white to black) ratio of suicidal deaths at age 80.

In two of the studies of 100 or more consecutive, unselected suicides, it was shown that certain combinations of age, sex, and psychiatric diagnoses indicate degree of risk. For instance, as seen in tables 9.4 and 9.5, both Barraclough and Robins found that the highest incidence of suicide in their samples occurred among subjects of both sexes over the age of 45 diagnosed as having suffered from affective disorder, depressed phase. In Robins' sample, the risk for men with affective disorder, depressed phase increased dramatically after age 60 (5:1). Barraclough, on the other hand, found a similar increase in risk at age 65, but in women rather than in men (3:1).

In subjects diagnosed as having had alcoholism, sex appears to have more bearing

Table 9.4. Age at Death, Sex, and Diagnoses from a Study of 100 Suicide Subjects in England (3)

Age	Depression		Alcoholism		Miscellaneous		Not Mentally Ill	
	Men	Women	Men	Women	Men	Women	Men	Women
15–24	4	0	0	0	0	0	0	1
25–44	5	6	3	1	4	4	1	0
45–64	16	13	9	1	0	1	1	0
65+	5	15	0	1	3	2	2	2
Total	30	34	12	3	7	7	4	3
Mean ages	50	58	50.9	53.0				

Table 9.5. Age at Death, Sex, and Diagnoses from a Study of 134 Suicide Subjects in St. Louis (5)

Age	Affective Disorder		Alcoholism		Miscellaneous		Undiagnosed	
	M	F	M	F	M	F	M	F
20–29	2	0	2	0	1	0	1	0
30–39	4	0	6	2	3	1	3	0
40–49	6	5	11	1	2	0	2	1
50–59	5	8	6	2	1	1	4	1
60–69	21	3	3	0	2	2	2	1
70+	7	2	0	0	5	0	4	1
Total	45	18	28	5	14	4	16	4
Mean age	58.5	54.9	45.8	44.4	56.5	53.0	55.1	59.5
Youngest	29	40	24	32	29	31	27	41
Oldest	86	72	62	56	85	63	85	80

on the degree of risk than does age. Robins found a ratio of between 5 and 6:1, men to women, in the alcoholic subjects. Barraclough's ratio was 4:1, men to women. Even so, age, especially in men, does seem to play a significant role. Robins' suicide study shows 45 as the mean age at death for alcoholic subjects in contrast with ages 58.5 for subjects with affective disorder. (Indeed, the difference in the modal ages is even greater—approximately 20 years). The age influence is harder to evaluate in Barraclough's figures because of his use of 20-year steps.

Communication of Intent

The authors of the three comprehensive suicide studies are in basic agreement on the question of what threatening suicide means in terms of eventually committing suicide. Barraclough et al (3) found that 55% of their sample had given clear indications of suicidal intent. Robins et al (5) found that 69% of their sample communicated suicidal intent, and Dorpat and Ripley (4) reported that 83% of their Seattle suicides had given direct and indirect warnings of suicidal intent. These findings would seem to deflate the old bromide, "If they talk about it, they won't do it."

Suicide Attempts as Predictors

Contrary to common opinion, suicide attempts are not ironclad predictors of completed suicide. Barraclough and his group (3) found that 30% of their subjects had made previous attempts; Dorpat and Ripley (4) found 33%; Robins et al (5) found 18%.

It is known that there is, among women, a somewhat higher percentage of attempters than among men and that multiple attempts, when they occur, occur more frequently among women than among men.

There have been several important studies—by von Andics and Ettlinger, among others—indicating the overlap in attempted and completed suicide and that that overlap occurs in "two directions," that is, that a certain percentage of attempters complete suicide (Ettlinger's (2) finding is about 1%/year) and that a somewhat higher percentage of completed suicides is preceded by attempts.

Antecedent Circumstances as Predictors

Among alcoholics who commit suicide, loss of affectional relationships—divorce or separation from a spouse; death of a spouse; bereavement involving the death of another relative or close friend; and other losses such as being left behind by a relative's move from home—plays a more important role than it does among those with depression. It was found, in the St. Louis study, that during the last year preceding suicide, 33 subjects (25% of the total sample) suffered the loss of an affectional relationship. Sixteen of these losses were experienced by subjects diagnosed as having alcoholism (or 48% of the alcoholic subjects as opposed to 14% of those with affective disorder); 11 of the 16 (33% of alcoholism subjects) occurred within 6 weeks of the suicidal event. In that last 6-week period, there were only two (3%) such losses in the affective disorder group.

It is possible that the higher number of affectional losses among the alcoholics throughout the last year of life is a result of chronicity of alcoholism and the difficulties involved in living with such chronically ill people. In contrast, affective disorder, as an illness, usually occurs in infrequent episodes that are not chronic and thus not so apt to lead to separation.

Another circumstance commonly thought to be associated with suicide is physical illness. However, as noted earlier, suicide is rare among people with *terminal* medical illness. It is interesting that Dorpat and Ripley's suicide study (4) showed that, of the 80 subjects about whom they had medical information, 56 shared a total of 107 illnesses. These 107 illnesses were categorized as 47 psychosomatic illnesses (including 17 peptic ulcers, 11 cases of hypertension, 12 cases of rheumatoid arthritis, and 7 unspecified illnesses), 16 cases of cardiovascular and heart disease, 6 malignancies, and 38 unspecified illnesses. Barraclough et al (3) reported that 5 of their 100 subjects had suffered from terminal medical illnesses—2 malignancies and 3 nonmalignant illnesses. In the St. Louis study, medical illness occurred in 61 of the 134 subjects (46%) and did not occur at the time of suicide in 63 subjects (47%). (The other 10 subjects were those on whom medical information was scant). There were an additional 10 subjects (7%) about whose physical health there was no information. In the study, informants were asked to judge relevant antecedent circumstances as "important," "questionably important," or "not important" in precipitating the suicides. The most commonly cited antecedent circumstance considered by the informants to be "important" to suicide was the occurrence of nonpsychiatric (medical) illness (5). Thus, while the prevalence of physical illness in suicide subjects in two of these studies was about 50%, the incidence of terminal medical illness in suicide subjects was, in contrast, 5% or less.

The other most common antecedent circumstances considered by the St. Louis informants to have been "important to the suicide" were, in order of prevalence, heavy drinking, friction with spouse or lover, job troubles, divorce or separation, financial difficulties, drinking just prior to suicide, and feelings of disgrace. Less common were friction with a close relative, death of a close relative, and sickness of a relative. Living alone, death of a close friend, sickness of a close friend, pregnancy, moving to another house, and having legal problems were cited as being "important" much less often. Occurring, but never cited as "important," were moving to another city, school problems, and, finally, situations in which no problems were known.

BEFORE SUICIDE

It is probable that the only generally effective means of reducing the suicide rate is to hospitalize suicidal patients in *closed wards*. To judge by the data of the St. Louis suicide study, two large subgroups of potentially suicidal patients are recognizable as such: those suffering from a depressive illness who communicate their suicidal intent and those with chronic alcoholism who communicate suicidal intent. These two subgroups constitute 49% of the total group of 134 suicides.

This finding suggests that, when a person in either of the above two subgroups comes to the attention of a physician, the physician should recommend immediate hospitalization in a closed psychiatric ward. Before physicians should accept this suggestion as a practical recommendation, however, they would need to know the answer to one further question: How many persons with these two diseases communicate suicidal ideas and do not commit suicide, even though they are not hospitalized? That is, how many persons would physicians hospitalize who did not, in fact, require hospitalization in order to prevent their suicides? The answer to this question is not known.

As far as depressive patients are concerned, it should be pointed out that there are, of course, reasons for hospitalization other than potential suicide. These include malnutrition, weight loss, ill advised decisions regarding marital, work, and social lives, and marked agitation. A study by Cassidy et al (9) suggests that about 25% of manic-depressive patients make such ill advised decisions regarding their lives during their illnesses (9). It is likely, therefore, that few patients are hospitalized without justification since, as pointed out above, there are a number of compelling reasons other than the prevention of suicide for hospitalizing depressive patients.

The difficulties of recommending closed ward hospitalization for all depressives who have communicated their suicidal intentions are obvious. However, hospitalization of all those patients might nevertheless be usefully considered for the following reasons. First, the St. Louis study results suggest that the elderly male depressive patient who has communicated his suicidal intentions is an especially serious suicide risk and that perhaps, at the very lest, all of these patients require hospitalization. Second, there are five studies (10) which indicate that an average of 14.5% of at least once hospitalized patients with depression will kill themselves in one or another depressive episode.

There are indications that the possibility of preventing suicide in manic-depressive patients may be better than in chronic alcoholics: manic-depressives receive more medical and psychiatric care, have a discrete, episodic illness with a marked and relatively acute behavior change highly visible to concerned relatives; have a short lived (months) illness with the prospect of a spontaneous (or induced) remission in the vast majority of instances; and are generally much more amenable to the necessity of closed ward hospitalization than are alcoholics.

Is education of the general public concerning the symptoms of affective disorder, depressed phase, part of the answer to the prevention of suicide? In the urban St. Louis area, 73% of those suicide subjects diagnosed as having had affective disorder, depressed phase, went to a physician for their symptoms within 1 year of their suicides. This is a high proportion of the cases and suggests that public education is less needed than are better criteria for hospitalization of such patients when they do see physicians. However, in St. Louis, for 20% of the affective disorder, depressed phase patients, hospitalization was recommended and not accepted by the relatives; therefore, public education along these lines must be considered.

Alcoholism presents a different problem. Although its symptoms are recognized by the general public, only 40% of these patients in the St. Louis study had medical or psychiatric care within 1 year preceding their suicides (5). This low proportion of alcoholics seen by physicians is probably related to the chronicity of the disease and to the isolation of advanced alcoholics from their families.

Finally, if it had been found that suicide was an impulsive, unpremediated act, then the problem of its prevention using presently available clinical criteria would present insurmountable difficulties. The high rates of communication of suicidal ideas found by all three of the studies of 100 or more suicides (3–5) indicate that in the majority of instances it *is* a premeditated act of which the person gives ample warning. Therefore, there is currently available to the physician information that he needs to take an active role in preventing suicide. To take this role, he must be able to diagnose the two illnesses from which the majority of the potential suicides are suffering, and he must insist on a careful history from the family and from the patient as to whether suicidal ideas have indeed been communicated.

SUMMARY

In the three studies of 100 or more suicides (3–5), investigators' findings emphasized the very high rate of mental illness among those who commit suicide—93 to 100%. Two illnesses—affective disorder, depressed phase, and alcoholism—account for the majority (54 to 85%) of psychiatric diagnoses in all of the studies. The percentage of persons who committed suicide who were *not* diagnosed as having suffered from a mental illness was low—0 to 7% of the total samples. It was found also that among the suicide subjects there was a high degree of need for medical care within the last year of life. In the St. Louis study, 73% of the subjects were under doctors' care in that year (5); in the Seattle study, Dorpat and Ripley reported 87% of their sample sought medical care in that year; and, in Britain, Barraclough et al found that 100% of their subjects sought the care of a physician in the final year, 40% within the last week prior to suicide and 19% within the last month, whereas only 7% of the controls in that study visited a doctor or underwent medical treatment in a given week (3).

These results indicate very clearly the association of mental illness and suicide, especially depression and suicide. It is encumbent upon physicians to recognize the symptoms of clinical depression and upon psychiatrists to recognize the need for hospitalization.

If diagnosis, referral, treatment, and necessary hospitalization are called for in suicide prevention, so are gun control and public education about the dangers of alcoholism and drug abuse. The most urgent need, however, is for further research on affective disorder and alcoholism, especially their biological aspects.

References

1. von Andics M: *Uber Sinn und Sinnlosigkeit des lebens.* Vienna, Gerold and Company, 1938.
2. Ettlinger RW: Suicides in a group of patients who had previously attempted suicide. *Acta Psychiatr Scand* 40:363–378, 1964.
3. Barraclough B, Bunch J, Nelson B, Sainsbury P: A hundred cases of suicide: clinical aspects. *Br J Psychiatry* 125:;355–373, 1974.
4. Dorpat TL, Ripley HS: A study of suicide in the Seattle area. *Compr Psychiatry* 1:349–359, 1960.
5. Robins E, Murphy GE, Wilkinson RH Jr, Gassner S, Kays J: Some clinical considerations in the prevention of suicide based on a study of 134 successful suicides. *Am J Public Health* 49:888–899, 1959.
6. Murphy GE, Robins E: Social factors in suicide. *JAMA* 199:303–308, 1967.
7. Shaffer JW, Perlin S, Schmidt CW Jr, Stevens JA: The prediction of suicide in schizophrenia. *J Nerv Ment Dis* 150:349–355, 1974.
8. *Leading Components of Upturn in Mortality for Men, United States—1952-67.* Vital and

Health Statistics Series 20, no. 11, Department of Health, Education and Welfare Publication no. (HSM) 72-1008. Washington, DC, US Government Printing Office, 1971.

9. Cassidy WL, Flanagan NB, Spellman M, Cohen ME: Clinical observations in manic-depressive disease. A quantitative study of one hundred manic-depressive patients and fifty medically sick controls. *JAMA* 164:1535–1546, 1957.

10. Guze S, Robins E: Suicide and primary affective disorders. *Br J Psychiatry* 117:437–483, 1970.

10

Suicide in Adolescents

Keith Hawton, D.M., M.R.C.Psych.

INTRODUCTION

Considerable concern has been expressed about the apparent recent increase in suicides among adolescents, particularly in the United States. Suicide in young people results in horror and disbelief, especially among relatives and friends of the deceased, and it is often the subject of sensational reports in the media. In view of the highly emotive responses to this problem it is important for professional workers concerned with adolescents to examine very carefully what facts are known about adolescent suicide.

In this chapter the more important aspects of this phenomenon are considered, including its epidemiology, possible causes, the likely reasons for the recent increase in the number of adolescent suicides, and prevention. Most emphasis will be on 10- to 20-year-olds, although reference will be made to children and young adults.

EPIDEMIOLOGY

Before examining recent trends in suicide among adolescents, some of the methodological problems encountered in obtaining accurate suicide statistics must be explored. These bedevil the study of suicide in all age groups but are especially pertinent when considering suicide among young people.

It is generally accepted that official suicide statistics underestimate the true rate of suicide. Various estimates of the extent of underreporting have been provided by studies in different countries. Thus it has been suggested that official suicide figures may represent between a quarter and two-thirds of the actual numbers of suicides (1–3). Several factors may contribute to these serious discrepancies. First, the criteria necessary for a verdict of suicide may be too stringent and may also vary between different countries. Second, the nature of other verdicts available to officials may encourage underreporting. For example, in the United Kingdom the verdict of undetermined cause of death will often be used where there is any doubt about the cause of death. Third, the officials who make such verdicts vary between different countries (e.g., medical officers in the U.S., coroners in England and Wales). Fourth, willingness to reach verdicts of suicide may be influenced by prevailing religious beliefs. Thus in Roman Catholic countries there may be great reluctance to attribute deaths to suicide.

There may be even greater underreporting of suicides among adolescents because the relative rarity of such events in this age group makes those responsible for determining the cause of death unlikely to consider suicide as an explanation. Furthermore, there may be considerable pressure to protect other individuals, especially parents, from the distress likely to be caused by a verdict of suicide in a young person.

All of these points should be borne in mind when considering the following suicide statistics.

Recent Trends

United States

Recent statistics for suicide in young people in the U.S. are summarized in Tables 10.1 and 10.2. The rates for 20- to 24-year-olds are included for comparison. Suicide rates among 15- to 19-year-olds of both sexes increased substantially between 1960 and 1981, the overall increase being 142% (similar increases occurred among 20- to 24-year-olds). In 1981, suicide was the third leading cause of death in this age group, behind only accidents and homicide (4, and personal communication regarding earlier reports). In terms of actual numbers of deaths by suicide in 1981 there were 1413 boys and 357 girls.

The marked increase in deaths by older teenagers between 1960 and 1981 occurred against a background of only a small (13%) increase in the suicide rates for all ages, much of which would have been accounted for by the increase among the young.

Suicide rates among 10- to 14-year-olds increased only slightly between 1960 and 1981 and were always much lower than among 15- to 19-year-olds (Tables 10.1 and 10.2). In terms of actual numbers, 115 boys and 48 girls in this age group died by suicide in 1981.

According to official figures, deaths by suicide are rare under the age of 10 years. For example, in 1981 only four such deaths were recorded, all boys.

Table 10.1. Male Suicide Rates in the U.S./100,000*

Year	Age Groups (Years)		
	10–14	15–19	20–24
1960	0.9	5.6	13.7
1965	0.9	6.1	16.3
1970	0.9	8.8	19.3
1975	1.2	12.0	25.9
1980	1.2	13.8	26.8
1981	1.2	13.6	25.6

* From Statistical Resources Branch, National Center for Health Statistics, United States Department of Health and Human Services, Washington, DC.

Table 10.2. Female Suicide Rates in the U.S./100,000*

Year	Age Groups (Years)		
	10–14	15–19	20–24
1960	0.2	1.6	2.9
1965	0.1	1.9	4.2
1970	0.3	2.9	5.7
1975	0.4	2.9	6.7
1980	0.3	3.0	5.5
1981	0.5	3.6	5.6

* From Statistical Resources Branch, National Center for Health Statistics, United States Department of Health and Human Services, Washington, DC.

United Kingdom

Recent suicide statistics for England and Wales are shown in Tables 10.3 and 10.4. Under 15-year-olds have been omitted from these tables because the numbers of deaths are so few (see below) that the rates are very unstable. Again, suicide statistics for 20- to 24-year-olds have been included for comparison.

Suicide rates for both boys and girls aged 15 to 19 increased during the mid-1960s (confirmed by year-on-year rates) and then declined toward the end of that decade (when, it should be noted, detoxification of the gas supply was taking place). Toward the end of the 1970s the rates again rose. Judging from the statistics available for the 3 years 1981 to 1983, there appears to have been a recent marked decline in suicide rates among females in this age group. However, the variations in rates over time for older teenagers in the United Kingdom are very small compared with recent changes in the U.S., where, in all years shown in Tables 10.1 to 10.4, the rates have been higher than in the United Kingdom.

The numbers of official suicides among children and adolescents under 15 years of age are small, having averaged around five per year since the early 1940s. There has, however, been a small decline in the rates for boys and a corresponding increase in the rates for girls.

A recent review of death statistics by McClure (5) suggests that the official suicide statistics in the United Kingdom have concealed the true picture of suicide in the young. Between 1951 and 1980 there was a substantial increase in deaths due to poisoning in the 10 to 14 age group which were categorized as "undetermined" or "accidental." Comparison of the decades 1951 to 1960 and 1971 to 1980 revealed a 5-fold increase in the numbers of such deaths. Similar trends occurred in these categories of deaths among 15- to 19-year-olds. It is common practice in the U.K. to

Table 10.3. Male Suicide Rates in England and Wales/100,000*

Year	Age Groups (Years)	
	15–19	20–24
1960	3.0	8.6
1965	4.3	8.8
1970	3.2	8.6
1975	3.4	9.6
1980	4.1	9.0
1983	4.0	9.6

* From Office of Population Censuses and Surveys, London.

Table 10.4. Female Suicide Rates in England and Wales/100,000*

Year	Age Groups (Years)	
	15–19	20–24
1960	1.5	3.8
1965	1.8	3.7
1970	1.4	3.7
1975	2.1	3.6
1980	2.0	4.1
1983	1.2	3.3

* From Office of Population Censuses and Surveys, London.

add undetermined deaths and accidental deaths due to poisoning and liquids to the official suicide figures to create an "estimated" suicide figure (6). When McClure (5) did this and then compared the change in the estimated suicide rate between 1968 to 1970 and 1978 to 1980 he found a marked increase for boys (+56%) and girls (+66%) in the 10- to 14-year age group, and for girls aged 15 to 19 years (+63%), and a less marked rise for boys aged 15 to 19 years (+21%). The changes for individuals of all ages were, by comparison, very small (males +7%; females −1%).

These findings suggest that the actual suicide rate among adolescents in the U.K. may have increased more substantially in recent years than is indicated by official statistics. Although there is likely to be a very real difference in suicide rates between the U.K. and the U.S., this discrepancy might be less than official figures suggest, because of the greater extent to which self-poisoning is used for suicide in the U.K., firearms and hanging (which cause less doubt as to intention) being far more popular in the U.S. (see below).

Sex, Race, Marital and Occupational Status

Sex

It can be seen from Tables 10.1 to 10.4 that suicides of young males outnumber those of females by a factor of between two and three. This contrasts with nonfatal suicidal acts, especially self-poisoning, where the situation is reversed (except in the very young). Thus the female-to-male ratio for attempted suicide by teenagers has been variously reported as being between 3:1 and 9:1 (7–9). The situation with regards to actual suicide in adolescents reflects the pattern found in adult suicides.

Race

Marked racial differences in suicide statistics are found in the U.S. Suicide is more common among white than nonwhite teenagers (Table 10.5). Although the ratio of the rates for teenagers and young adults in these two groups decreased to almost parity around 1970, a very marked increase in rates among whites during the 1970s meant that by 1980 the ratio was almost 2:1 (4).

These findings are difficult to explain, especially since unemployment, poverty, alcoholism, and other risk factors for suicide are more common among young blacks. It has been suggested that a greater tendency to outwardly directed aggression among

Table 10.5. Suicide Rates of Young Whites and Nonwhites in the U.S./100,000*

| | Age Groups (Years) | | | | | |
| | 10–14 | | 15–19 | | 20–24 | |
	White	Nonwhite	White	Nonwhite	White	Nonwhite
Males						
1960	1.0	0.2	5.9	3.4	11.9	7.8
1970	1.1	0.3	9.4	5.4	19.3	19.4
1980	1.4	0.4	15.0	7.5	27.8	20.9
Females						
1960	0.2	0.0	1.6	1.5	3.1	1.6
1970	0.3	0.4	2.9	2.9	5.7	5.5
1980	0.3	0.1	3.3	1.8	5.9	3.6

*From Statistical Resources Branch, National Center for Health Statistics, United States Department of Health and Human Sciences, Washington, DC.

blacks reduces the risk of both depression and suicidal behavior, but this is not compatible with the facts that antisocial behavior is a common precursor of childhood suicide, and depression is common among delinquent adolescents (10). Another possibility is that, although blacks probably face more social stresses than do whites, suicidal behavior might be less socially sanctioned among blacks than among whites. This requires investigation. Furthermore, blacks might also have more effective social support systems, a possibility which is consistent with the relatively low suicide rates found in young blacks reared in traditional southern states settings compared with those of young blacks living in the northern states, who are more likely to have been subject to deculturalization (10).

Suicide rates are particularly high among North American Indians and apparently are increasing in all age groups (11). Among 15- to 24-year-olds the rates are 5 times those of the general population. However, the rates vary quite considerably between different Indian reservations and appear to be correlated with the prevalence of social problems (12).

Marital Status

Suicides are more common among married than single teenagers, the ratio of the rates in married individuals to those in single persons in the 15- to 19-year age group being approximately 1.5 for males and 1.7 for females (13). This is in marked contrast to the situation in adults where suicide is less common among married people than among those who are single or divorced (14). The most likely explanation is that teenage marriages are often forced by pregnancy or are hastily established as a means of escaping from an unhappy home environment and are hence likely to encounter major difficulties.

Unemployment

Little appears to be known about the effects of unemployment on suicide rates among older teenagers, although the association between suicide and unemployment in adults is well documented (15, 16). Common sense and the recognized increased risk of mental ill health among young people who are unemployed (17) suggest that a similar association should apply in the young. This is a most important question in view of the recent steep rise in unemployment rates among young people in many western countries. It is also possible that any current increased risk will eventually decline as unemployment becomes more widely accepted and the unemployed therefore feel less stigmatized.

University Students

Suicide among university students has attracted considerable attention, probably because of the wastage of potential that such suicides represent and the responsibility that universities have in terms of caring for the mental health of their students and preventing suicides. Consistent and quite remarkable transatlantic discrepancies have emerged from studies of suicide in students, with a considerably increased risk being found among students in the United Kingdom compared with general population suicide rates, but no such difference being found in the U.S. The U.K. studies have primarily focussed on students at Oxford and Cambridge Universities. Extremely high rates were reported for such students during the period 1945 to 1955 (18). A more recent study by the author demonstrated an increased risk of suicide among Oxford University students compared with the general population of similar age for the period

1966 to 1976, although the risk was not as great as found in the earlier studies (19). By contrast, the risk for attempted suicide was much less among the students than among other young people.

In North America, much lower rates of suicide have been found among students at Yale and Harvard Universities compared with their British counterparts (20, 21)—the risk of suicide at these universities and at other American universities being similar to that in the general population of the same age (13). Indeed, students at Alberta University in Canada were found to have a lower suicide rate than expected from general population figures (22).

These transatlantic differences are difficult to explain. One possibility is that particularly severe stresses might be faced by Oxbridge students, although this seems unlikely, especially when compared with students at Yale and Harvard. Another is that the selection policy at the U.K. universities might allow entry to students at particular risk of psychological instability into an environment which for some can result in extreme isolation. It should be noted, however, that the risk of suicide at Oxford in recent years appears to have declined, suggesting that any causal factors are now less significant. A major recent change of possible significance in this respect (23) has been a very considerable reduction in the ratio of male to female students attending the university.

Methods Used for Suicide

Marked international differences are found in the predominant methods used in suicides by young people, which probably reflect differences in availability of the various means. In the U.S., for example, firearms are the predominant method, whereas they are relatively rarely used in the U.K. (Table 10.6). By contrast, suicides due to "poisoning by liquids and solids" (mostly overdoses) are far more common in the U.K. than in the U.S. A further indication of the extent to which availability influences the method chosen for suicide was the finding among adolescents in Ontario

Table 10.6. Methods Used in Suicides by Adolescents in the U.S. (1981) and in England and Wales (1983)*

	Age Groups (Years)				
	10–14†	15–19		20–24	
	U.S.	U.S.	E and W	U.S.	E and W
	%	%	%	%	%
Firearms	52.9	66.0	5.9	62.7	9.4
Hanging, strangling, and suffocation	32.0	18.0	29.4	15.6	27.7
Poisoning by liquids and solids	12.8	2.2	23.5	7.7	22.7
Poisoning by gas	0.6	7.8	5.9	6.3	18.8
Other	1.7	5.9	35.3‡	7.8	21.5‡

* From Statistical Resources Branch, National Center for Health Statistics, United States Department of Health and Human Services, Washington, DC; Office of Population Censuses and Surveys, London.

† The figurees for 10- to 14-year-olds in England and Wales were omitted because of small numbers.

‡ Jumping from high places was common among the "other" methods in England and Wales.

where firearms were more commonly used in rural areas, and drugs and jumping from heights more often in urban areas (9).

Domestic gas used to be a popular means of suicide in the U.K., but suicidal deaths by this means decreased steadily as the gas supply was detoxified during the 1960s. None of the deaths due to poisoning by gas in England and Wales in 1983 (Table 10.6) were the result of domestic gas poisoning, most involving motor vehicle exhaust gas.

There are also marked sex differences in the methods used for suicide by adolescents, males tending to use violent means (e.g., firearms, hanging) and females to use poisons. This has been related to higher aggressiveness among males, although differential availability of means is also likely to be important. For example, males are most likely to have experience with and access to firearms, whereas females are more likely to be prescribed psychotropic drugs.

CONTRIBUTORY FACTORS

Considerable difficulties are encountered when one tries to examine the cause of suicide, especially in the young. The major problem stems from the necessarily retrospective nature of such investigation. The usual method is to carry out what has been termed a "psychological postmortem," in which information used to establish a profile of the dead person is gathered from several sources, such as relatives and friends, and medical and other files. The data from such an examination of several individuals are then pooled in order to identify typical features of suicides and to delineate subgroups. This type of study has virtually never been conducted on sizable groups of adolescent suicides. A notable exception was the very detailed study of 30 suicides, aged 12 to 14 years, which was conducted in the U.K. by Shaffer (24). One reason for the paucity of this type of investigation in adolescents is the distress that it is likely to cause informants, especially relatives of the dead person.

A further difficulty in retrospective studies of suicides is that the information will often be collected many months or years after death. Important information, such as that concerning an individual's personaltiy, mental state, and intellectual level, may have gone unrecorded. Furthermore, the recollection of informants may have been distorted by the passage of time and the effects of the suicide.

Because of these problems one must try to analyze as carefully as possible the information that is available concerning possible contributory factors. A useful first step is to separate such factors into those which are predisposing to suicide and those which appear to precipitate the fatal act.

Predisposing Factors

Family Background

It might be thought that adolescents who kill themselves, as with their adult counterparts (25), would often be from either broken homes or families in which there is an unhappy relationship between the parents. In Shaffer's study (24), 7 of the 30 young adolescent suicides had experienced broken homes by the time they died, and in 6 cases the parents separated within 4 years following the suicide. In a study of a large group of young suicides in Sacramento County, California, half of the individuals had experienced "loss or family disruption" by the time of their death (26). However, these figures are no greater than would be expected among psychiatrically disturbed children in general. This is surprising in view of the association between attempted suicide among adolescents and broken homes and unhappy family backgrounds (8, 9,

27). It might be explained by the fact that although loss or separation of parents is easy to identify in retrospect, other evidence of parental difficulties may be far less accessible than in prospective investigations (which are more feasible when studying attempted suicide).

Some information is available concerning psychiatric disorder and suicidal behavior among first-degree relatives of adolescents who kill themselves. In Shaffer's study (24), four first-degree relatives had a history of suicide attempts, and three made attempts after the adolescents' suicides. This proportion of adolescents with a family history of an attempt is comparable with that found in adolescents who make nonfatal attempts. This might reflect a relatively high incidence of psychiatric disorder, especially depression, in such families. Suicidal behavior by relatives might occasionally also provide a model of coping for an adolescent.

Psychiatric Disorders

In spite of the difficulties inherent in retrospective identification of psychiatric disorders in young people, such disorders appear to be relatively common. For half the sample in Shaffer's study (24) there was evidence of some type of psychiatric disturbance, with antisocial symptoms (e.g., bullying, stealing, truancy) and emotional symptoms (depression, excessive fears or school refusal) being equally common. In their study in Sacramento County, California, Cosand and colleagues (26) found evidence of "emotional instability" in a third of their 15- to 19-year-old suicides, 17% of this group having received psychiatric treatment. Garfinkel and Golombek (9) reported that "significant psychiatric conditions" were recorded at the inquest or necropsy in a quarter of their adolescent suicides in Ontario, with depression being most common, but a substantial proportion having schizophrenia.

Such figures are much lower than those reported for adult suicides: for example, Barraclough and colleagues (28) identified psychiatric disorders in 93% of their cohort, the vast majority having suffered from depression. It seems likely that although psychiatric disorder is often an important factor in adolescent suicide, external circumstances may be equally important.

Physical Illness

Although physical disorders are common among adult suicides, especially the elderly, they rarely appear to be a major contributory factor in adolescent and child suicides, particularly in the very young (26). However, a physical illness, even though minor, might constitute a predisposing factor rendering the individual more vulnerable than usual to distress caused by social factors.

Previous Suicide Attempts

There is a very important association between completed suicide and nonfatal suicidal behavior. As many as 40% of young suicides will have a history of a previous attempt (10, 26). Few long term follow-up studies of adolescent suicide attempters have been conducted, so that the risk of eventual suicide is unclear. In a Swedish investigation of 1547 adolescent suicide attempters, 4.3% had died by suicide during the 10- to 15-year follow-up period (7), whereas only 0.24% of 2492 adolescent self-poisoners studied in the U.K. had died in this way during a follow-up period which averaged 2.8 years after the initial overdoses (29). This discrepancy may be due to two factors. First, the Swedish study included self-injuries as well as overdoses, and the risk of suicide is greater in the former. Second, the U.K. study was conducted almost

20 years after the Sweidsh study, during which time there had been a vast increase in the incidence of self-poisoning, probably because of a disproportionate increase in the numbers of adolescents making less serious attempts who were therefore at less risk of subsequent suicide.

Both studies, however, were in agreement that the risk of eventual suicide is greatest among males, especially older teenage boys.

Precipitants

Suicide does not necessarily follow a clear precipitant. Suicidal ideation will often develop gradually, especially when it is the result of an increasing sense of hopelessness consequent upon depression. In many cases, however, a clear external precipitant will be apparent. In Shaffer's (24) group of 30 adolescent suicides aged 10 to 14, 36% of the fatal acts appeared to follow a disciplinary crisis. Some of the individuals had been told by a teacher at school that their parents were about to be informed of truanting or other antisocial behavior, and the others were anticipating either punishment at school or a court action. Less common precipitants were disputes with peers, parents, or a boyfriend or girlfriend. Interestingly, three individuals had a psychotic parent, and all had expressed distress at having to live with the mad parent; two of the suicides occurred on the day when the parent was due to be discharged from a psychiatric hospital. Bereavements were possible contributory factors in six cases, although the time relationship between the deaths, all of which involved family members, and the suicides were not clear.

Antecedents of suicide in older adolescents have not been as clearly documented as in Shaffer's study. It is likely that becoming unemployed, disruption of the relationship with a partner, and threatened conviction might be some of the more important.

The nature of the precipitants of suicide is likely to vary according to the social environment, a major stress in one setting being less significant in another because of differences in expectation. This is illustrated by the situation in Japan, which has extremely high rates of suicide among the young, where it has been suggested that the intensely stressful preparation for the national college entrance examination, the outcome of which virtually decides an individual's future, is a major factor (30).

A further factor, which is discussed in more detail below, concerns the reporting of suicide by the media. There is now ample evidence that such reports are often followed by an increased number of further suicides (31).

POSSIBLE REASONS FOR THE INCREASE IN SUICIDE AMONG THE YOUNG

During the past two decades there undoubtedly has been an increase in suicide among adolescents, especially among older teenagers and particularly in the U.S. One can only speculate about likely contributory factors, the causes almost certainly being multifactorial. Obvious factors to be examined include major changes in the social environment, altered attitudes toward suicide, increased availability of means for suicide, and changing patterns of psychopathology.

Changes in the Social Environment

Vast social changes which are likely to be relevant to suicide in the young have occurred during the past two or three decades. One has been the loosening of family ties, particularly as a result of the vast rise in divorce rates. The increased risk of both depression and suicide in people who have experienced death of a parent during childhood is well documented (32, 33). Whether loss through separation is such a potent factor is unclear. However, loss of family supports is becoming increasingly common, and often occurs at an early age. This has coincided with young people having to face pressures of adulthood earlier in life. For example, sexual relationships are often established in early adolescence, with the risk of considerable distress following their disruption. Evidence is now available demonstrating the importance of supportive relationships at such times, and how depression is a likely consequence when these are not available (32).

A further change has resulted from the threat of nuclear war, which has been present to varying and generally increasing degrees during the past 30 years. The knowledge that existence has become so precarious might facilitate the development of hopelessness in the face of other adversities.

Changing Attitudes toward Suicide

Suicide rates tend to correlate with the degrees of acceptance of suicidal behavior in particular cultures. This is exemplified by the situation in Japan, where suicide has historically been viewed as an acceptable and sometimes even honorable option, and where very high suicide rates prevail. By contrast, suicide rates in predominantly Roman Catholic countries, in which suicide is regarded as sinful, tend to be relatively low. Evidence of less negative recent attitudes to suicide is not easy to obtain. However, weakening of religious faith has occurred throughout much of the western world, and it is possible that inhibitions on suicide may have decreased as a result of this.

Another factor which is likely to influence attitudes to suicide is the way in which it is discussed in the media. Such discussions are increasingly common. Furthermore, it is now apparent that media reports of suicides can facilitate suicides by other people. For examle, Barraclough and colleagues (31) demonstrated a statistical association between reports of suicides in a local newspaper and the subsequent suicides of men aged under 45. Other studies confirming the facilitatory effect of publicity on suicides have been reported (34, 35).

In view of the extensive publicity which often follows suicides by young people, such a factor might operate particularly powerfully in adolescents. In the U.S. there has been a recent concern that a media-related contagion effect might have contributed to the increased number of suicides involving older teenagers. An example of a cluster of suicides which attracted particular attention occurred in Plano, Texas, where there were seven suicides among 15- to 18-year-olds between February 19 and August 22, 1983 (36). Some of the suicides were clearly linked. Thus, two of the boys were friends, and another boy was found to have newspaper clippings concerning two of the suicides displayed in his room. A further cluster of adolescent suicides occurred in Westchester County, New York, at the beginning of 1984, when there were five suicides during 3 weeks (36). The victims were not acquainted with each other, but the suicides received considerable attention in the local media.

It is possible that such clusters occur purely by chance. However, the connections between some of the individuals in the first example, and the empirical evidence from investigations of the patterns of suicides following newspaper reports of suicidal deaths, make this explanation less likely. Assuming that there is a facilitatory effect of media reporting of suicides, this phenomenon requries explanation. Straightforward imitation seems unlikely, although it is well recognized that the means employed in suicide may be copied from the published suicidal deaths of others. The outbreak in Britain of suicide by burning following a couple of widely publicized deaths of this kind, for example (37). A more likely explanation of how media reporting might facilitate suicide is that some individuals who are entertaining suicidal ideas may be encouraged to act on them through reading about the suicides of others. A further possibility is that the knowledge that publicity will result might also encourage a person to act in this way, especially when revenge constitutes part of the motivation for the act.

Increased Availability of Means of Suicide

The most common methods of suicide used in a given area or country usually reflect availability. The use of firearms for suicide in the U.S. provides one example, and coal-gas suicides in the U.K. prior to detoxification of the gas are another. Altered availability is only likely to result in an increase in suicides if an acceptable and reliable method becomes more widely available. More widespread availability of firearms to young people in the U.S. is an obvious example. The recent increase in the use of mood-altering medication might be another. The widespread prescribing of tranquilizers and antidepressants, often in response to requests for help for social problems rather than psychiatric disorders, may have resulted in altered attitudes to their use, both as a means of dealing with stress and as a means of obtaining oblivion, either temporary or permanent. While part of the increase in young suicides may be attributed to this factor, this is not consistent with the evidence that females are more likely both to receive psychotropic drugs and to take them in overdose, but the sex ratio for completed suicide (more males than females) is the reverse of that in attempted suicide. Furthermore, in the U.K. there was a decline in the rates of official suicide verdicts during the late 1960s and early 1970s, the very time when nonfatal self-poisoning became very much more common than previously.

Changing Patterns of Psychopathology

A further possibility is that psychiatric disorders in young people are becoming more common. The author knows of no evidence to support this idea. However, the increase in the numbers of young persons who now experience broken homes, and in the other stresses encountered by young people today, suggests that this may have occurred. There is more substantial evidence for a recent increase in drug addiction and alcoholism among the young, both of which carry a high risk of eventual suicide.

PREVENTION OF SUICIDE

The question of how to prevent young suicides can be considered in two parts: First, general measures which might reduce the risk of suicide; and second, the management of the suicidal adolescent once he or she has been identified.

General Methods of Prevention

Suicide Prevention Centers

In recent years there has been considerable enthusiasm for suicide prevention and crisis intervention centers in both the U.K. (where the Samaritan organization is especially well known) and the U.S. This enthusiasm has been countered by controversial and contradictory research findings concerning the role of such centers in actually preventing suicides. In Britain, for examle, Bagley (38) reported evidence of a decline in rates of suicide in cities in which branches of the Samaritan organization had been established and an increase in rates in matched cities which did not have Samaritan branches. However, a subsequent replication of this study, in which the authors claimed to have included control cities which were better matched with the cities with Samaritan branches than those in Bagley's study, failed to support the earlier finding (39).

In the U.S., two investigations of suicide prevention centers failed to demonstrate any substantial preventive effect (40, 41). On the other hand, a recent study has been more encouraging, especially with regard to prevention of suicide among young people (42). While little difference in changes in overall suicide rates was found between counties in which crisis information centers were established between 1968 and 1973 and those which lacked such centers during this period, a significant difference was found between them for suicides by white females under 24 years of age. Thus there was a decline in suicide rates of 55% in counties in which crisis centers were established and an increase of 85% in those in which they were not. This finding was replicated for a different set of counties for a different time period. The validity of this finding is enhanced by the knowledge that young white females are the most frequent callers at crisis centers. The authors suggested that more than 600 lives/year might be saved if suicide prevention centers were generally available throughout the U.S.

Reduced Availability of the Means of Suicide

The extremely wide availability of many means of suicide might suggest that trying to reduce their availability is pointless. However, many suicidal acts are impulsive and rely on the immediate availability of a method, and even in individuals with serious suicidal intent, one method may be acceptable while others are not. Furthermore, many individuals are extremely ambivalent about going through with a suicidal act (43). Therefore, measures which require serious consideration include reducing the availability of guns, especially in the U.S., and of psychotropic agents and nonprescribed analgesics. Many household medicine cabinets are stocked with medicines no longer needed but often dangerous in overdosage. Educating people to store only medicines which are absolutely necessary, and then to keep them in relatively small quantities, might help to prevent some fatal overdoses.

Reduced Publicity about Suicides

The evidence concerning the facilitatory effect of media publicity on suicides strongly suggests that serious efforts should be made to encourage newspapers and other forms of media to restrict this form of publicity, especially where young people are involved, perhaps only reporting the essential facts and in as undramatic a fashion as possible.

Provision of Advice on Coping Strategies

Some schools now allocate time in their curricula for discussion of problems young people are likely to face and appropriate coping strategies. In general this seems a sensible move, and it might help to prevent some suicides, especially if advice is given on ways of obtaining help when adolescents are faced by overwhelming stress.

Management of the Suicidal Adolescent

Many adults who commit suicide have been in contact with potential helping agencies shortly beforehand (28). Although little information is available about such contacts by adolescent suicides, half of a series of adolescents who took nonfatal overdoses had consulted their family doctor during the month before their overdoses (8). Smaller proportions had been in contact with either social work or psychiatric agencies. Thus, prevention of suicidal acts is theoretically feasible in many cases. Furthermore, young people particularly at risk of suicide are those who have already made suicide attempts and those with major psychiatric disorders, especially depression. Such individuals will also usually have come to the notice of potential helping agencies.

There is, however, a major statistical problem in suicide prevention, even when those at risk have been recognized. The criteria that might help in the detection of those most at risk are crude, applying to many more individuals who will not kill themselves than those who will. Therefore, it is not sensible to consider suicide prevention in isolation, but far better to plan the management of depressed and suicidal adolescents in general, with the primary aim being amelioration of social and psychological problems, and the secondary aim that of occasionally preventing suicide. However, this should not discourage professionals from using their knowledge of those factors which predict an increased risk of suicide to identify individuals who may require special attention.

Assessment

Professionals who encounter adolescents in distress are adivsed to take seriously any threats of suicide, however vague these might appear. When depression or suicidal ideas are accompanied by a sense of hopelessness, this is a particularly important warning sign. Suicidal ideas should never be condemned, but should be acknowledged and then carefully explored, especially with regard to possible suicidal plans. There is no evidence to support the fear that inquiry about suicidal ideas might encourage a suicidal act. Rather, it is likely to allow identification of individuals most at risk and hence facilitate prevention.

Detection of depression in adolescents is often more difficult than in adults, especially in the very young in whom psychosomatic complaints are sometimes a primary manifestation. Other major psychiatric disorders associated with risk of suicide, such as schizophrenia, are usually more obvious.

In addition to exploration of suicidal ideas, a thorough assessment of the distressed and/or suicidal adolescent should include inquiry about the following:

1. Family history, especially of parental separation, bereavement, psychiatric disorder, and suicidal behavior;
2. Previous psychiatric disorder;
3. Previous suicide attempts;
4. Current problems—especially regarding school/work, family, boy/girlfriend, legal or financial difficulties, alcohol, and drugs;
5. Potential sources of support (e.g., family, friends, or professional helpers) and the individual's willingness to use them.

When an adolescent is seen following a suicidal attempt, the inquiry should also include an estimate of the degree of suicidal intent. This requires information about the circumstances of the act (premeditation, planning, isolation, suicide note), the person's stated intention, and his or her attitude about having survived. A persistent sense of hopelessness when little immediate change in the circumstances can be expected should be taken very seriously. A full description of assessment procedures for young people who have made suicide attempts is available elsewhere (44).

Treatment

A major psychiatric disorder and/or immediate risk of suicide will often be an indication for admission to an adolescent psychiatric unit. However, most adolescents with psychiatric disorders can be managed as outpatients. During the period of greatest distress it is most important to ensure that a supportive individual whom the young person appears to trust is readily available. Many crisis intervention services have an "open access" or "hot line" facility whereby it is possible for an individual to telephone the agency if facing intolerable stress. Adolescent affective disorders appear to respond just as well to physical treatments, such as antidepressant therapy, as do equivalent disorders in adulthood. However, psychological therapies will be the mainstay of treatment. Family therapy is the treatment of choice for many young adolescents and for some older adolescents who have not yet separated either physically or psychologically from their parents. Individual counseling will often be more appropriate for older adolescents, a problem-solving approach (45) providing a useful model. There is a need to explore the use of cognitive therapy in suicidal and depressed adolescents, particularly in view of its usefulness for these conditions in adults (46).

CONCLUSIONS

In recent years suicide has undoubtedly become a major problem among adolescents, especially older teenagers, particularly in the U.S. Some possible explanations for this have been explored in this chapter. Further research into this problem is urgently required. For example, there is considerable need for an extensive investigation of a large series of adolescent suicides, painful as this type of research might be. The psychological postmortem approach should be employed, which necessitates obtaining information from several sources, including family members, professionals who knew the adolescents before their death, and school and hospital documents. Such a study should provide far more detailed profiles of adolescents who kill themselves than it has been possible to provide in this chapter on the basis of research to date.

A recent finding from the U.S. suggests that suicide prevention schemes might be effective in young people. This should encourage further efforts into making helping agencies more widely available for adolescents. Other possible means of prevention include reducing media publicity concerning young suicides, reducing the availability of some of the methods used for suicide, providing time in school curricula to discuss problem-solving skills, and adequately identifying, assessing, and treating adolescent psychiatric disorders.

References

1. Dublin LJ: *Suicide: A Sociological and Statistical Study.* New York, Ronald, 1963.
2. Ovenstone IMK: A psychiatric approach to the diagnosis of suicide and its effect upon the Edinburgh statistics. *Br J Psychiatry* 124:315–321, 1973.
3. McCarthy PD, Walsh D: Suicide in Dublin. I. The under-reporting of suicide and the consequences for national statistics. *Br J Psychiatry* 126:301–308, 1975.
4. National Center for Health Statistics: *Monthly Vital Statistics Reports* 33(3), 1981.
5. McClure GMG: Recent trends in suicide amongst the young. *Br J Psychiatry* 144:134–138, 1984.
6. Adelstein A, Mardon C: Suicides 1961–74. In *Population Trends*, no. 2. London, Her Majesty's Stationery Office, 1975, p 13.
7. Otto U: Suicidal acts by children and adolescents. *Acta Psychiatr Scand* (Suppl 233), 1972.
8. Hawton K, O'Grady J, Osborn M, Cole D: Adolescents who take overdoses: their characteristics, problems and contacts with helping agencies. *Br J Psychiatry* 140:118–123, 1982.
9. Garfinkel BD, Golombek H: Suicidal behaviour in adolescence. In Golombek H, Garfinkel BD (eds): *The Adolescent and Mood Disturbance.* New York, International Universities Press, 1983, p 189.

10. Shaffer D, Fisher P: The epidemiology of suicide in children and adolescents. *J Am Acad Child Psychiatry* 20:545–565, 1981.
11. U.S. Department of Health, Education, and Welfare: *Suicide, Homicide, and Alcoholism among American Indians: Guidelines for Help.* Publication no. (ADM) 74-42. Rockville, MD, Department of Health, Education, and Welfare, 1973.
12. McCarney ER: Adolescent and young adult suicide in the United States—a reflection of societal unrest? *Adolescence* 14:765–774, 1979.
13. Petzel SV, Cline DW: Adolescent suicide: epidemiological and biological aspects. *Adolesc Psychiatry* 6:239–266, 1978.
14. Kreitman (ed): *Parasuicide.* London, John Wiley & Sons, 1977.
15. Platt S: Unemployment and suicidal behaviour: a review of the literature. *Soc Sci Med* 19:93–115, 1984.
16. Sainsbury P: *Suicide in London.* London, Chapman and Hall, 1955.
17. Banks MH, Jackson PR: Unemployment and risk of minor psychiatric disorder in young people: cross-sectional and longitudinal evidence. *Psychol Med* 12:789–798, 1982.
18. Carpenter RG: Statistical analysis of suicide and other mortality rates of students. *Br J Prev Soc Med* 13:163–174, 1959.
19. Hawton KE, Crowle J, Simkin S, Bancroft, J: Attempted suicide and suicide among Oxford University students. *Br J Psychiatry* 132:506–509, 1978.
20. Parrish HM: Epidemiology of suicide among college students. *Yale J Biol Med* 29:585–595, 1957.
21. Elsenberg L: Adolescent suicide: on taking arms against a sea of troubles. *Pediatrics* 66:315–320, 1980.
22. Sims L, Ball MJ: Suicide among university students. *J Am Coll Health Assoc* 21:336–338, 1973.
23. Cresswell PA, Smith GA: *Student Suicide: A Study in Social Integration.* Cambridge, private publication, 1968.
24. Shaffer D: Suicide in childhood and early adolescence. *J Child Psychol Psychiatry* 15:275–291, 1974.
25. Dorpat TL, Jackson JK, Ripley HS: Broken homes and attempted suicide. *Arch Gen Psychiatry* 12:213–216, 1965.
26. Cosand BJ, Bourque LB, Kraus JF: Suicide among adolescents in Sacramento County, California 1950–1979. *Adolescence* 17:917–930, 1982.
27. Jacobs J: *Adolescent Suicide.* New York, Wiley-Interscience, 1971.
28. Barraclough B, Bunch J, Nelson B, Sainsbury P: A hundred cases of suicide: clinical aspects. *Br J Psychiatry* 125:355–373, 1974.
29. Goldacre M, Hawton K: Repetition of self-poisoning and subsequent death in adolescents who take overdoses. *Br J Psychiatry* 146:395–398, 1985.
30. Igu M: Suicide of Japanese youth. *Suicide Life Threat Behav* 11:17–30, 1981.
31. Barraclough B, Shepherd D, Jennings C: Do newspaper reports of coroner's inquests incite people to commit suicide? *Br J Psychiatry* 131:528–532, 1977.
32. Brown GW, Harris T: *Social Origins of Depression.* London, Tavistock, 1978.
33. Bunch J, Barraclough BM, Nelson B, Sainsbury P: Early parental bereavement and suicide. *Soc Psychiatry* 6:193–199, 1971.
34. Phillips DP: The influence of suggestion on suicide: substantive and theoretical implications of the Werther effect. *Am Sociol Rev* 39:340–354, 1974.
35. Bollen KA, Phillips DP: Imitative suicides: a national study of the effects of television news stories. *Am Sociol Rev* 47:802–809, 1982.
36. *Washington Post*, March 11th, 1984.
37. Ashton JR, Donnan S: Suicide by burning as an epidemic phenomenon: an analysis of 82 deaths and inquests in England and Wales in 1978–1979. *Psychol Med* 11:735–739, 1981.
38. Bagley C: The evaluation of a suicide prevention scheme by an ecological method. *Soc Sci Med* 2:1–14, 1968.
39. Jennings C, Barraclough BM, Moss JR: Have the Samaritans lowered the suicide rate? A controlled study. *Psychol Med* 8:413–422, 1978.

40. Weiner IW: The effectiveness of a suicide prevention program. *Ment Hyg* 53:357–363, 1969.
41. Lester D: Effect of suicide prevention centers on suicide rates in the United States. *Health Services Rep* 89:37–39, 1974.
42. Miller HL, Coombs DW, Leeper JD, Barton SN: An analysis of the effects of suicide prevention facilities on suicide rates in the United States. *Am J Public Health* 74:340–343, 1984.
43. Eisenberg L: The epidemiology of suicide in adolescents. *Pediatr Ann* 13:47–54, 1984.
44. Hawton K: *Suicide and Attempted Suicide in Adolescents and Children.* Beverly Hills, CA, Sage, in press.
45. Hawton K, Catalan J: *Attempted Suicide: A Practical Guide to Its Nature and Management.* Oxford, Oxford University Press, 1982.
46. Beck AT, Rush AJ, Shaw BF, Emery G: *Cognitive Therapy of Depression.* New York, Guilford, 1979.

11

Suicide and Physical Illness

F. A. Whitlock, M.D., F.R.C.P., F.R.C.Psych.

On commonsense grounds one might expect many persons with chronic, painful or terminal illnesses to end their suffering prematurely by taking their own lives. In fact, such rational decisions to commit suicide are relatively rare. It follows, therefore, that unless a physical illness brings on a severe depression, the great majority of patients will die naturally rather than predetermine their ends. Such an assumption is well supported by mortality statistics. In elderly persons, among whom chronic painful illnesses are common, suicide accounts for only 0.5% of male and 0.2% of female deaths. Because other causes of death are less frequent in younger subjects, suicide constitutes a far higher percentage of deaths than in those aged more than 60 years.

This is not to deny that considerable numbers of persons of all ages who commit suicide have autopsy and inquest evidence of physical disease. The figures given in Table 11.1 indicate the varying extent of this association which to some degree will depend on the thoroughness with which the investigations were carried out and recorded. Nonetheless, the existence of physical diseases cannot be taken as incontrovertible evidence that illness was the sole or even the most important factor leading to suicide. To take one example, in the study by Chynoweth and co-workers (1), where postmortem findings were particularly complete, physical illness was found in more than half of the victims. In nearly half of this group (47%) alcoholism and/or barbiturate dependence was almost certainly a contributory factor, and at least 40% were severely depressed. From such observations it would be difficult to argue that physical illness alone was the determinant of suicide, although in one-quarter of the whole sample it was considered to be the principal factor.

Although it has been stated repeatedly that physical illness and suicide are strongly associated with one another, few investigations have included adequate controls with whom to compare the suicide data. Specific diseases, such as epilepsy, malignant neoplasms, and gastrointestinal and musculoskeletal disorders, appear to occur more frequently in suicide victims than would be expected. Unless these observations are carefully matched with those from a control population, one cannot say with absolute certainty that these physical conditions exceed what one would find in the general community. This, of course, does not invalidate the opinion that physical illness can be a major cause of suicide in some diseases, of which epilepsy is a prime example. Many disorders will precipitate severe depression, but in some cases of suicide it is reasonable to conclude that this choice of death was a rational act. For example, a 56-year-old man died following a drug overdose. One year previously he had undergone a total cystectomy and subsequently required a tube and bag to collect his urine. He also suffered from severe pain from a recurrence of a carcinoma in his throat. Finally,

152 / *Suicide*

Table 11.1. The Prevalence of Physical Illness in 15 Studies of Suicides

Place	No. of Suicides	No. with Physical Illness
Brisbane, Australia, 1973–1974 (1)	135	70 (52%)
London, 1955 (2)	390	113 (29%)
Seattle, 1960 (3)	80	56 (70%)
Keighley, U.K., 1952–1959 (4)	122	85 (70%)
Shropshire, U.K., 1965–1972 (5)	256 Psychiatric patients	76 (30%)
West Sussex, U.K., 1966–1967 (6)	30 aged 65+	17 (57%)
Helsinki, 1952–1963 (7)	57 Psychiatric patients	18 (31.6%)
United States 1959–1966 (8)	630	171 (27%)
Brisbane, Australia, 1935–1940 (11)	184	46 (25%)
St. Louis, 1956–1957 (12)	134	62 (46%)
Bristol, U.K., 1957–1961 (13)	325	65 (20%)
Lund, Sweden, 1962 (14)	46 Psychiatric patients	21 (45.6%)
Brisbane, Australia, 1965 (15)	165	29 (18%)
Brighton, U.K., 1963–1969 (16)	170	84 (49%)
England and Wales, 1968–1970 (present study)	1000	363 (36%)

Total suicides (excluding psychiatric and geriatric patients) = 3338
Total with physical illness (excluding psychiatric and geriatric patients) = 1144
(34.3%)

4 months before his death, total removal of his external genitalia was carried out because of another cancerous growth. Not surprisingly the coroner considered his death to be the almost inevitable outcome of intolerable suffering. A diagnosis of depression in such a case seems to be superfluous to the needs of the verdict.

In many follow-up reports on specific diseases one encounters sporadic instances of suicide or, more frequently, attempted suicide during the course of the illness. For obvious reasons, if the patient had taken his life early on in his illness before coming for treatment he would not be included in the follow-up account of survivors. This sets limits to the extent to which one can argue with complete assurance that a particular physical illness has a higher than expected rate of suicide as a cause of death. Consequently, one must turn to well controlled postmortem findings to ascertain the true situation. Even then, however, one other factor is almost invariably omitted—the effects of treatment. There is abundant evidence that many drugs in common use today can cause severe depression and suicidal behavior. The likelihood that this contribution to a suicide death will be elicited by a coroner's inquiry is small as, almost certainly, the disease for which drugs were being administered will take priority as the most probable cause of the victim's death. The frequency of drug-induced depression leading to suicide is not known, although the liability to such disasters is greater with patients who have past personal histories of affective disorders.

THE EPIDEMIOLOGY OF SUICIDE AND PHYSICAL ILLNESS

Figures from 15 reports (Table 11.1) show that the prevalence of physical illness in suicides varies from 25 to 70% of cases and that it appeared to be an important contributory cause of the patient's death in 10.9 to 51%. Sainsbury (2), in his well known study of suicide in London, estimated that malignant neoplasms occurred 20 times more often than expected. Tuberculosis and parkinsonism were respectively 10 times and 200 times more prevalent than in the general population. Dorpat and Ripley (3) in Seattle found particularly high rates of physical illness in their suicide sample (70%) and considered that in 41% of cases this was a major factor contributing to the suicide's death. In their series cancer was 15 times, rheumatoid arthritis 5 to 7 times, peptic ulcer 2 to 5 times, and hypertension 2 to 3 times more common than the expected rates of these diseases in the general population. Stewart (4), a pathologist, provided autopsy findings on 122 cases of suicide. Only 37 (30%) were free from disease, but it is difficult to assess the suicidal significance of the physical disorders in the other 85 victims. Nonetheless, one might conclude that some cases of peptic ulcer, five cases of malignant neoplasm, one case of advanced multiple sclerosis, and one possible case of Cushing's syndrome were severely depressed and suicidal.

When investigations are restricted to special groups of patients the same high prevalence of physical illness is found. Myers and Neal (5), for example, observed that 30% of 256 psychiatrically ill patients were physically ill before committing suicide. They noted the higher incidence of suicide among epileptic patients with schizophrenic-like psychoses and that 6.2% of their patients had definite evidence of organic brain disease diagnosed during life. A further 10 who had not been so diagnosed before their deaths were found to have cerebral atrophy at autopsy. Barraclough (6) limited his investigations to 30 cases of suicide aged more than 65 years old. Physical illness was present to a significant degree in 17 (56%), a finding which was considerably greater than in a matched control group who had sustained accidental deaths.

Stenback and co-workers (7) also reported their findings on psychiatric patients who had committed suicide. Physical illness was found in 31.6% of those in hospital compared with 36.4% of nonhospitalized patients. On the other hand, physical illness was present in 40.5% of nonsuicidal psychiatric patients. Hence it was concluded that, so far as psychiatric patients are concerned, the prevalence of physical illness is no greater in the suicidal than in the nonsuicidal. Farberow and colleagues (8) investigated the extent of psychiatric and physical illness in 630 cases of suicide. The great majority had been suffering from psychiatric disorders, but there appeared to be an excess of those with malignant neoplasms and cardiovascular and respiratory diseases. For these two last groups, however, this excess was not statistically significant.

As might be expected, all investigators have reported higher rates of physical illness in elderly suicides. For example, Gatter and colleagues (9) found that among 1862 suicides the frequency of physical illness among male victims rose from 6.25% for those aged less than 45 years old to 50.2% for those aged over 65 years. For females the rates were 5.9% and 32.9%, respectively, for these two age groups.

An investigation of the prevalence of physical illness among 200 suicides compared with a matched sample of accident victims showed a significant excess of physical disease in the suicide sample (Table 11.2). Only in the group aged 40 to 59 years old was there a statistically significant increase of physical disease affecting the female but not the male suicides. In the other two age groups the excess of suicides with physical disorders was not statistically significant. In both sexes, whether they died accidentally or by suicide, there was a steady increase in the numbers with physical illness from the youngest to the oldest age group. This study of a relatively small number of cases generally supports the opinion that more suicides are physically ill compared with nonsuicidal members of the community. On the other hand, the increase is not as great as might be expected, largely on account of the mounting incidence of disease in older persons, regardless of their modes of death.

Table 11.2. Physical Illness in 200 Suicides and 200 Accident Deaths Based on Autopsy Findings in Brisbane, 1970 to 1975

	No. with Physical Illness	
	Suicides	Accident Deaths
Ages 20 to 39 (males 53, females 17)	Males 7 (13.2%)	Males 1 (1.9%)
	Females 1 (5.9%)	Females 1 (5.9%)
Ages 40 to 49 (males 55, females 34)	Males 25 (45.4%)	Males 22 (40%)
	Females 20 (58.8%)	Females 10 (29.4%)
Ages 60+ (males 23, females 18)	Males 14 (60.9%)	Males 10 (43.4%)
	Females 12 (66.7%)	Females 8 (44.4%)

In each sample: total males 131, total females 69

Male suicides with physical illness = 46 (35.1%)
Female suicides with physical illness = 33 (47.8%)
Male accident deaths with physical illness = 33 (25.2%)
Female accident deaths with physical illness = 19 (27.4%)
Male suicides versus accidents $\chi^2 = 2.88$ (not significant)
Female suicides versus accidents $\chi^2 = 9.8$ ($p < 0.005$)
Ages 40 to 49 female suicides versus accidents $\chi^2 = 4.83$ ($p < 0.05$)
All suicides versus all accidents $\chi^2 = 8.27$ ($p < 0.005$)

One Thousand Suicides in England and Wales

Few investigations of physical illness affecting suicide victims have compared their findings with the estimated prevalence of various medical and surgical illnesses in the general population. To overcome this deficiency, information was obtained on 1000 suicides recorded in 20 coroners' districts over the years 1968 to 1972 (to be referred to throughout this chapter as the EWTS study). The demographic data and number with physical illness in this cohort are given in Table 11.3, and diagnostic details recorded in the coroners' reports are listed in Table 11.4.

Because many of the suicides were suffering from more than one disease before their deaths, the total number of diseases and symptoms (473) is considerably greater than the number of persons afflicted with physical illness (363). Inevitably there has been some duplication, an example being the three cases of cerebral tumor also listed under the heading of cancer. This, in turn, will include some of those who had recently received surgical treatment. In some cases it might be assumed that the figures represent minimal findings because most information on physical disease wsa derived from the pathologists' reports, which would not comment on symptoms such as chronic pain and visual defects. In some cases pain would have been the consequence of arthritis and other physical disorders whose nature was not specified at the time of the inquests. A percentage of those suffering from chronic ill health almost certainly would have been troubled by conditions given under separate headings, but, unfortunately, the exact nature of the ill health mentioned in these reports was not recorded. Consideration of the individual conditions listed in Table 11.4 will be deferred to the appropriate sections of this chapter when particular physical diseases will be discussed.

Table 11.5 compares the observed numbers of selected diseases affecting the suicide victims with the same illnesses in the general population. The latter data were obtained from the *Morbidity Statistics from General Practice, 1971–1972* (10) from which the prevalence rates were estimated for the three age groups, 15 to 44, 45 to 64 and 65 and over. The numbers in each age group in the suicide population were used as the basis for estimating the number of patients in the General Practice survey who would have been suffering from the same diseases. The statistical significance of the observed compared with the expected numbers is derived from Poisson distribution tables.

Diseases of the Central Nervous System

Because of the increased incidence of major depression in patients with cerebral disease, the association of suicide with such illnesses is hardly surprising. High on the list of brain disorders causing suicide are epilepsy, multiple sclerosis, brain damage following head injuries, cerebrovascular disease, Huntington's chorea, and progressive organic deterioration leading to dementia. Other conditions, such as paralysis agitans,

Table 11.3. 1000 Suicides in England and Wales (EWTS)

	Ages			
	15–44	45–64	65+	Total
Completed suicides				
Males	170	222	150	542
Females	113	192	153	458
Persons	283	414	303	1000
Suicides with physical illness				
Males	31 (18.2%)	89 (40.1%)	82 (54.7%)	202 (37.3%)
Females	31 (27.4%)	58 (30.2%)	72 (47.0%)	161 (35.1%)
Persons	62 (21.9%)	147 (35.5%)	154 (50.8%)	363 (36.3%)

Table 11.4. Physical Diseases, etc in EWTS Study

Disease	No.	Disease	No.
CNS disease		Pregnancy, etc	6
Epilepsy	25	Cardiovascular disease	
Multiple sclerosis	6	Cardiac disease	33
Cerebrovascular disease	27	Hypertension	24
Dementia	11	Vascular disease	7
Head injuries	9	Respiratory disease	
Tumors	3	Asthma	13
Leukotomy	4	Chronic bronchitis and	19
Miscellaneous	5	emphysema	
Visual defect	14	"Influenza"	14
Deafness	3	Tuberculosis	12
Gastrointestinal disease		Pleurisy	1
Active peptic ulcer	26	Musculoskeletal disorders	
Healed peptic ulcer	24	Arthritis	39
Partial gastrectomy	22	Pain	13
Hepatic cirrhosis, diseases of	4	Other locomotor disabilities	15
gallbladder and pancreas		Endocrine diseases	
Other bowel disease	5	Diabetes	8
Cancer	32	Thyroid dysfunction	4
Recent surgery	33	Genitourinary disease	26
Pending surgery	4	Chronic ill health	20
Anemia	6	Other conditions	2
Skin disease	4		

Total disease, etc (*less* healed peptic ulcer, gastrectomy, and pending surgery) = 473

Table 11.5. Prevalence of Physical Illness in 1000 Suicides (EWTS) Compared with General Practice Consultations (1971 to 1972) (MSGP)

		Ages			
		15–44	45–64	65+	Total
Epilepsy	EWTS	13*	11*	1	25†
	MSGP	0.9	1.4	0.9	3.2
Epilepsy (males)	EWTS	6‡	7‡	0	13*
	MSGP	0.5	0.7	0.5	1.7
Epilepsy (females)	EWTS	7*	4‡	1	12*
	MSGP	0.4	0.6	0.3	1.5
Cerebrovascular disease	EWTS	1	10	16	27*
	MSGP	0.07	1.9	8.5	6.2
Dementia	EWTS		1	10*	11*
	MSGP		0.1	1.6	0.9
Visual defect	EWTS		2	12	14*
	MSGP		1.1	4.3	3.2
Multiple sclerosis	EWTS				6*
	MSGP				0.76
Head injury	EWTS				9‡
	MSGP				1.4
Cerebral tumor	EWTS				3*
	MSGP				0.12
Peptic ulcer (active)	EWTS	11	9	6	26†
	MSGP	1.3	3.5	1.6	5.9
Peptic ulcer (males)	EWTS	8	7	5	20*
	MSGP	1.2	2.8	3.8	4.0
Peptic ulcer (females)	EWTS	3	2	1	6
	MSGP	0.24	0.9	0.5	3.2
Cancer	EWTS	0	13*	19*	32†
	MSGP	0.3	3.7	6.3	6.7
Cardiac disease	EWTS	2	12	19	33
	MSGP	0.8	14.7	36‡	31.9
Hypertension	EWTS	1	12	11	24
	MSGP	1.4	16.6	20.6	26
Bronchitis	EWTS	0	7	12	19
	MSGP	0.85	9.1	12.2	14.9
Asthma	EWTS	3	6	4	13
	MSGP	2.3	3.8	2.4	9.7
Arthritis	EWTS	1	11	27	38
	MSGP	3.9	23.3	34	43
Endocrine diseases	EWTS				12
	MSGP				10.2
Anemia	EWTS				6
	MSGP				11.9
Cirrhosis, etc	EWTS				4‡
	MSGP				0.62
Surgical operation	EWTS				33
	MSGP				21.7

* $p < 0.01$.
† $p < 0.001$.
‡ $p < 0.05$.

are well known to cause serious depression, but death by suicide amongst patients suffering from this condition is unusual.

Epilepsy

Epilepsy appears to be one of the few conditions capable of causing suicide without the patient experiencing a period of severe depression beforehand. Cases have been recorded (17, 18) where a sudden urge of suicidal feelings occurred as part of an ictus. Older writers (19, 20) referred to suicidal insanity or mania, which in all probability, in some cases, was epileptic in origin. On the other hand, severe depression, either as an ictal or postictal phenomenon, may cause some patients to contemplate or actually to commit suicide. Barraclough (21) has reviewed 11 papers on epileptic suicide and found the ratio of observed to expected deaths to be about 5:1. Amongst temporal lobe epileptics the rate of suicide is 25 times greater than would be expected. Given a prevalence of epilepsy of between 3.5 and 5.5/1000 of the general population in the United Kingdom, the number of cases in the EWTS study is between 4.5 and 7.1 times greater than the general prevalence rate, a finding which is in keeping with the figures in Barraclough's report.

In the U.S., 5% of epileptic deaths were suicides, compared with 1.4% of deaths in the general population (22). In a table of suicide deaths among epileptics the frequency varied from 2.2 to 9.3%. An English investigation recorded increased deaths among epileptics from suicide and cancer of the central nervous system, the ratio of observed to expected suicide deaths being 5.4:1 (23).

Many other studies, most of which have been summarized by Barraclough, demonstrate this increased suicide mortality amongst epileptic patients, although the rates amongst institutionalized patients are lower than those of epileptics living in the community.

Apart from ictal and postictal depression some epileptic suicides will probably occur in a setting of psychosis or in response to what the patient perceives as an intolerable condition in which social restrictions and the unpredictable nature of the attacks may play a part. These factors may contribute to the higher rates of suicide among younger epileptics who may also be suffering from temporal lobe foci more often than patients with seizures developing later in life. This higher rate of suicide amongst early onset epilepsy was noted by Zielinski (24), who found that the risk among females was twice that of males. Similar findings emerged from the EWTS study, where the rate for females aged 15 to 44 (61.9/1000) was almost twice that of males in the same age group (35.3/1000).

Multiple Sclerosis

Faced by the prospect of lifelong, progressive disability with ultimate confinement to a wheelchair, double incontinence, and recurrent urinary tract infections, it is surprising that suicide among multiple sclerosis sufferers is a relatively rare event—a further indication that what might be called rational grounds for taking one's life contribute only slightly to the frequency of suicide among patients with serious physical illnesses. Nonetheless, Kahana and colleagues (25) reported that 3% of patients with cerebral lesions took their own lives, a suicide rate which is 14 times greater than that prevailing in the general population in Israel. Severe depression is more likely to complicate cases of multiple sclerosis with cerebral involvement and may develop before neurological symptoms and signs appear (26). Taking the prevalence rate for multiple sclerosis as 0.4 to 0.8/1000 in Great Britain, the finding of 6 cases in the

EWTS study is very significantly greater than the number that would have been expected. Stewart's (4) series included one case, but none of the other investigations so far mentioned recorded any examples of multiple sclerosis among the other physical illnesses associated with suicide. In an investigation (27) of 30 multiple sclerosis patients at least one attempted to kill herself, and others admitted to harboring serious thoughts of committing suicide. One patient with manic-depressive psychosis, possibly induced by cerebral damage, finally committed suicide during a depressive episode.

Head Injuries

According to Lishman (28), suicide is very considerably increased among patients who have sustained head injuries, and, as might be expected, such deaths most commonly occur in a setting of depressive psychosis. Lewin and colleagues (29), in a long term follow-up of patients who had survived severe head injuries, reported 73 deaths, 3 of which were suicides. Although this is 3 times greater than the expected number, it is not a statistically significant difference. Possibly brain damage suffered in wartime, as in the Finno-Russian War, is more conducive to depression, alcoholism, and suicide than are civilian casualties. Achté and Anttinen (30) found that 14.2% of deaths among brain-damaged Finnish soldiers were suicides, and Vauhkonen (31) reported the same percentage among 260 deaths of men disabled by brain injuries. The longer the period of incapacity, the greater was the risk of suicide. Cases with damage to the frontal and temporal lobes predominated, but there were no significant hemispheric differences. The 9 cases with histories of head injury in the EWTS study significantly exceeded the expected number, but only 2 of Sainsbury's series were said to have suffered brain damage, a rate of 5/1000, which is not a statistically significant increase.

Apart from the cases of war injuries reported from Scandinavian investigations, the association between brain damage and suicide is not very strong. Nonetheless, the trend among civilian casualties is similar to the consequences of brain trauma in wartime, and an augmented risk of suicide among these patients should be remembered by those working in head injury rehabilitation centers.

Cerebrovascular Disease

Although suicidal thoughts and attempts have been reported among patients with basilar artery insufficiency (32), there is a paucity of data on actual suicides among patients who have suffered strokes or subarachnoid hemorrhage. Sainsbury (2) found 4 cases of cerebrovascular disease in his series of suicides, a rate of 10/1000. The 27 cases in the EWTS study had all sustained strokes, and probably some of those with hypertension would have had cerebral changes without having the added misfortune of a hemorrhage or infarction. Cerebrovascular disease occurs more often in the oldest section of the population but, accepting a prevalence rate of 4.5/1000 for all ages (33), Sainsbury and the EWTS study reveal figures which are 2.2 and 6.0 times greater than would be expected. Following strokes (34), subarachnoid hemorrhage (35, 36), and cerebrovascular disease in the elderly, depression is common enough, but the frequency of suicide among these patients is unknown. The evidence presented here suggests that among older patients the risk is high enough to justify early and effective treatment of depression when this develops.

Huntington's Chorea

Huntington (37) characterized the disease that bears his name as one "with a tendency to insanity and suicide," and many subsequent reports testify to this fact.

Although dementia, paranoid psychosis, and personality change are most often mentioned, there can be no doubt that severe depression, attempted suicide, and actual death by suicide are equally important features of the illness. In a study of 88 cases (38), 28 had major depressive disorders and 8 suffered from bipolar affective disorders. Twenty-six had attempted suicide or had suicidal thoughts. Suicidal behavior is more likely to occur early in the disease and becomes less frequent once the patient has been admitted to hospital (39). According to Chiu and Alexander (40) the rate of death by suicide amongst 182 deaths recorded between 1952 and 1979 was 1.6%. From these data one might infer that although suicidal behavior by patients with Huntington's disease is frequent, death by suicide is relatively uncommon. Probably this is because the majority of patients are in hospital under supervision where they die from natural causes. In contrast, Reed and Chandler (41) found that 7% of noninstitutionalized patients with Huntington's disease died by suicide. That there was no case of Huntington's disease in the EWTS survey is hardly surprising considering that in the United Kingdom the prevalence of this condition varies from 4.0/100,000 in Carlisle (33) to 6.3/100,000 in Northamptonshire (42).

Other Diseases of the Central Nervous System

Cerebral Tumors. Three cases of cerebral tumor among 1000 suicide victims is not a very large number, but it is considerably greater than the reported prevalence rate of 0.49/1000 (33) in Great Britain. Similarly, the 2 cases in Sainsbury's series (5.1/1000) substantially exceeded the expected number. Cerebral tumors are relatively uncommon neoplasms, but it has been claimed that 10% of cases give way to "suicidal tendencies" (43). Nonetheless, Keschner and co-workers (44) considered suicidal feelings among patients with brain tumors to be rare. The findings reported here suggest that although suicide may be an unusual termination to the course of brain cancer, it occurs more frequently than would be expected on the basis of the prevalence rate in the general population.

Dementia. Symptoms and signs of dementia develop in about 10% of persons aged 65 years and over, 20% of these being cases of multi-infarct dementia. The General Practice morbidity study (10) refers only to senile and presenile dementia, and consequently the findings from the EWTS survey are not comparable. All except 1 of the recorded cases were aged over 64 years, but of the other 10, only 2 cases were specifically stated to be suffering from senile dementia. Eight cases of probable multi-infarct dementia, therefore, are significantly fewer than would be expected.

Paralysis Agitans. In the EWTS study only one case of paralysis agitans was recorded, and he was also said to be suffering from arteriosclerotic dementia. According to Brewin and co-workers (33) the prevalence of parkinsonism in the general population is 1.14/1000. It follows, therefore, that there was no increase in the prevalence of this disease in the EWTS survey. One of Mindham's (45) 89 patients, however, said to have arteriosclerotic parkinsonism, took his life; and Schneider and colleagues (46), who conducted a 5-year follow-up investigation of 127 parkinsonian patients, reported 30 deaths, of which 3 were suicides. Such deaths were more often associated with a late onset of illness and more cerebro-organic involvement. Hence one might conclude that suicide, when it does occur in cases of Parkinson's disease, will be associated with severe depression and incipient dementia and should not be regarded as a reaction to a progressive and crippling disease. In this context it is worth mentioning Parant's (47) opinion in 1892 when he wrote: "One of the most common and serious symptoms of melancholic depression in paralysis agitans is the tendency to suicide which is found in the majority labouring under this affliction." Sainsbury estimated that the number of cases of Parkinson's disease among his suicides was 200 times greater than would be expected.

Cancer

All of the studies mentioned so far in this chapter have shown that in a cohort of suicide victims there is a very considerable excess of those suffering from malignant neoplasms; and to this rule the EWTS study is no exception. Table 11.6 shows the rates in five investigations.

Sainsbury estimated the cancer prevalence in suicide victims to be 20 times greater than in the general population, although Dorpat and Ripley (3), despite the higher rate in their sample, considered the prevalence to be only 15 times greater than the expected number. In the Brisbane study, of the three cases of malignancy, one had not been diagnosed before death, a finding relevant to an investigation comparing the prevalence of cancer in suicide victims with accident cases (48). Seventeen of the suicides had malignant tumors, compared with two in the control group. In seven of the suicides and one of the accident cases the diagnoses of malignancy had not been made until the tumors were discovered at autopsy.

An alternative way of examining the problem was shown by Fox and colleagues (49), who reported the frequency of suicide among patients on a tumor registry. The suicide rate was increased for men but not for women, with the frequency being greatest soon after the diagnosis had been made. Fortunately, this rate declined during the subsequent years of survival. A rather similar study (50) showed the rate of suicide in a cohort of cancer patients to be 1.3 times greater than the general male population rate and 1.9 times greater for females. The highest rates were found in patients with gastrointestinal cancer, but patients with nonlocalized disease were no more at risk than those with defined tumors. Furthermore, patients treated by chemotherapy rather than by surgery and radiotherapy were more likely to take their own lives.

In connection with this topic, it is well known that cancer phobia or delusional beliefs that one has cancer are not unusual symptoms of severe depression and may lead to suicide, possibly to forestall the diagnosis being made. At least 14 cases in the EWTS survey were said to have expressed fears of cancer, and no fewer than 5 of these cases had been diagnosed as suffering from endogenous depression. In 3 cases there was a past history of treated cancer which might have given some substance to the fears that afflicted these patients.

The question arises, why do patients with cancer have higher suicide rates than the rest of the population? Leaving aside those patients who develop a severe melancholia as part of the cancer syndrome, there can be no doubt that the diagnosis of cancer conjures up images of extreme pain and suffering, sufficient to precipitate a determined act of suicide. In some of the cases in the EWTS series there was evidence that severe, intolerable pain and major disabilities were responsible for the patients' decisions to put an end to their sufferings rather than wait for death which, in these cases, would

Table 11.6. Malignant Neoplasms in Suicide Victims

	No. of Cases	Rate per 1000
EWTS	32/1000	32
Brisbane (1)	3/135	22
London (2)	14/390	36
Seattle (3)	6/80	75
Keighley (4)	5/122	41

not have been long delayed. In such cases one might hope that effective control of pain and treatment of depression when this is present would set limits to the number of cases of suicide among those afflicted with cancer.

Gastrointestinal Diseases

The increased frequency of peptic ulceration among suicide victims has been demonstrated by a number of investigators, some of whose findings are summarized in Table 11.7.

These high rates of peptic ulceration among suicide victims are probably related to the prevalence of alcoholism as a cause of gastritis and ulceration of the upper gastrointestinal tract. Stewart (4) found that 2 of his 10 cases with peptic ulceration and gastritis had very severe hypertrophic gastritis, probably alcoholic in origin. Additional inducements to suicide in these cases could have been "nervous instability," pain, and fears of cancer and operation.

In addition to the 26 cases with active peptic ulceration in the EWTS study, there were 24 with past histories of illness and treatment. Twenty-two of these 50 cases had been treated by partial gastrectomy, a finding of relevance to an investigation (51) in which it was found that 14 of 25 patients who had been operated on in this manner were alcoholic or dependent on mainly barbiturate sedatives. One of these patients finally committed suicide. Krause (52) found that the suicide rate among patients whose peptic ulcers had been treated by partial gastrectomy or gastroenterostomy was 6.8 times greater than the expected number, while another investigation (53) showed that the ratio of observed to expected suicide deaths among surgically treated peptic ulcer patients ranged from 2.7 to 3.9:1. Knop and Fischer (54) stated that 13.7% of deaths among patients with duodenal ulcer treated by Billroth II resections were suicides. The ratios of observed to expected deaths were 4.3:1 for men and 5.4:1 for women, both statistically significant at the 0.1% level of probability. Ross and co-workers (55) also reported a significant increase ($p < 0.05$) in the number of suicides among patients whose peptic ulcers had been treated surgically. In the mainly European literature on this topic, gastric rather than duodenal ulcers were most commonly diagnosed in alcoholic patients (56), while a higher rate of gastrectomy was reported among alcoholic compared with nonalcoholic patients (57–60).

In the EWTS series the numbers with *active* peptic ulceration at the time of their deaths were significantly greater for males in all three age groups but only for females aged 15 to 44. With respect to the 22 cases who had been treated by partial gastrectomy, *at least* 8 were considered to have been alcoholics or dependent on barbiturates. Unfortunately, the data are insufficient to enable a more exact assessment of this issue to be made, but only 2 of the alcoholic and drug-dependent subjects had *not* received

Table 11.7. Peptic Ulceration among Suicide Victims

	No. of Suicides	Peptic Ulcer	Rate (%)	Ratio Observed/Expected
Seattle	80	17	21.2	2.5
Keighley	122	8	6.5	11.0*
London	390	15	3.8	6.4*
EWTS	1000	26	2.6	4.4*
Brisbane	135	3	2.2	3.7*
U.S.	630	8	1.3	

* Based on an expected rate of 5.9/1000 (General Practice morbidity study).

surgical treatment. The difference between these gastrectomized and nongastrecto-mized cases is statistically significant at the 5% level of probability. In the absence of information on the prevalence of patients in the community whose peptic ulcers have been treated surgically, one cannot estimate the significance of the number of such cases in the EWTS survey, although almost certainly it is in excess of the expected figure.

The work of others and the survey reported here suggest that, although the discom-forts and anxieties caused by active peptic ulceration may induce some patients to take their own lives, the role of alcoholism is probably the more important determinant of both physical disease and suicide. This is not the place to review the contribution of alcoholism and excessive drinking to suicidal behavior, as this is a well established and accepted fact. The excessive prevalence of peptic ulcers among suicide victims and higher rates of suicide among patients with this type of gastrointestinal disease strongly suggest that alcoholism and its consequential depression are the intermediate variables contributing to self-destruction by these patients.

Other Gastrointestinal Diseases. The figure of four cases of cirrhosis of the liver and gallbladder disease in the EWTS series is 6.4 times greater than would be expected, and Sainsbury's finding of 4 cases of hepatic cirrhosis is 16.5 times higher. Once again the role of alcohol is an important factor leading to suicide in these cases. Two cases in the Brisbane study had manifest liver disease, and one of these was an alcoholic. No doubt, the rising number of alcoholics and deaths from cirrhosis in Great Britain today ensure an increase in the number of suicides with liver disease compared with their prevalence 15 years ago.

Among the 5 cases with other types of bowel disease in the EWTS study was 1 with Crohn's disease. This was probably a coincidental finding, although Carney and Sheffield (61) reported a high incidence of serious depression and suicidal attempts in 10 patients suffering from this condition.

Urogenital Disease

Surprisingly little has been written on the effects of urogenital disease on mood and suicidal behavior, particularly in the male. Nonetheless, Pons (62), in 1892, wrote: "Affections of the bladder (cystitis, retention of urine, stone) frequently influence mental functions ... in some patients a tendency to suicide is observed." More recently, Fawcett (63) described a 50-year-old man who, following a transurethral resection of the prostate, made a number of serious suicidal attempts. This author considered urological surgery to be one of the commoner precipitants of depression in men, an opinion supported by a urologist (64) who commented on the frequency of depression in men with prostatism and the need for prompt psychiatric referral to forestall death by suicide. In fact, it is probably within the experience of most psychiatrists practicing in general hospitals to receive calls to urology departments to advise on patients who have become depressed. Dunlop's (65) investigation of a group of patients attending a urological clinic included children with enuresis and women seeking advice for infertility and for other gynecological problems. A greater incidence of depression was found among patients with lower than with upper urinary tract symptoms.

Of the 26 suicides in the EWTS study with known urogenital disorders, only 2 were women, omitting those with purely gynecological complaints. If one also excludes those with acute cystitis from the General Practice morbidity study (10), one finds a striking increase in men aged 65 years and over among the suicide sample. The majority were suffering from symptoms suggestive of prostatism or had recently undergone prostatectomy. Five men in this age group were suffering from cancer, but even when this number is removed, the increase in urogenital disorders among elderly men remains a statistically significant finding. This increase of urogenital disease did not appear in younger male suicides nor among women of any age group.

Two of Stewart's (4) cases had enlarged prostates, and one had recently undergone prostatectomy. Another man had been treated for cancer of the prostate by prostatectomy and cystectomy, as a result of which he was permanently incontinent. Five of the cases in the Brisbane study (1), one woman and four men, were suffering from a variety of urological disorders, but there was no obvious excess in any age or sex group. Nonetheless, the overall rate of 37/1000 is more than twice the number expected from the General Practice morbidity study.

The absence of age data from Stewart's investigation makes it impossible to say whether all three cases mentioned were in the oldest age group, but considering the nature of their diseases, this seems probable. This finding coupled with the results in the EWTS series seems to imply a need for careful follow-up of elderly men suffering from or being treated for urological complaints. One might speculate that pain, incontinence, loss of sexual capacity, and fear of surgery could all play parts in inducing depression sufficiently severe in some cases to end with suicide.

Dialysis and Renal Transplant.   In the context of urological disease it is important not to overlook the effects of dialysis and renal transplant because depression often develops in patients undergoing dialysis (66). In a survey of deaths among patients being treated by renal dialysis, 10 of 574 were suicides and an additional 26 could be classed as suicides because the patients stopped treatment or failed to follow advice on diet and other requirements for a successful outcome to treatment (67). This report from Switzerland estimated that the suicide rate among dialysis patients was 9 to 10 times greater than that prevailing in the general population. The reasons for suicide included impaired quality of life, loss of sex drive and potency, severe depression, and the generally high age of the patients being treated. In the U.S., Abrams and colleagues (68) estimated that suicide by dialysis patients was 100 times greater than that of nondialysis subjects. If those who stopped treatment or failed to follow the treatment program were included as suicides, the rate became 400 times greater than the expected number.

Cardiovascular Diseases and Hypertension

In the EWTS study the prevalence neither of cardiovascular disease nor of hypertension exceeded the expected numbers. Undoubtedly some of those suffering from cardiac disease would also have been hypertensive, as would some of the cases with cerebrovascular disorder, but the figures by themselves do not show any significant increase in diseases of the cardiovascular system among the suicides. In this respect the findings are not dissimilar from Sainsbury's, who found 15 cases with cardiovascular disease among his London suicides, a rate of 3.8%. On the other hand, 20% of the suicides in Seattle (3) were said to have had cardiovascular *and* heart disease (sic), and an additional 14% were hypertensive. The number of cases with hypertension was 2.8 times the expected figure. Stewart (4) gave details of 33 cases with hypertension and cardiac hypertrophy, but at least 20 also had other diseases. If this number is deducted, the 13 cardiac and hypertensive suicides in a total of 122 (10.6%) gives a figure intermediate between the London and Seattle findings. Farberow and co-workers (8) considered that, among their suicides, those with circulatory disease exceeded the number to be found in general medical and surgical hospitals, and a review of suicides in general hospitals (69) was of the opinion that depression leading to suicide occurred particularly in patients experiencing their first episodes of cardiac symptoms.

An important factor to be taken into account in some suicides suffering from hypertension and cardiac disease would be the effects of medication, as some drugs such as reserpine and methyldopa are well known causes of depression in a proportion of patients receiving this kind of treatment. On the other hand, the evidence on drug-induced depression suggests that patients who have had previous attacks of affective disorder are most at risk (70). From this conflicting evidence it would be difficult to reach a firm conclusion on the question of whether cardiovascular disease per se is a significant factor precipitating depression and suicide. Elderly men with higher suicide rates are also more likely to suffer from cardiac disease and hypertension, but the association of these phenomena in this age group may be purely coincidental.

Respiratory Disease

As was the case with cardiovascular disease, there was no significant increase in the prevalence of respiratory disorders among the suicides in the EWTS study. Chronic bronchitis and emphysema affected only the two older age groups, which is consistent with the greater prevalence of these disorders among older patients. Asthma, independent of bronchitis, was said to have been a distressing condition in 13 cases, but, again, this is not an excessive number compared with the overall prevalence of the disease. Fourteen cases were said to have suffered infections diagnosed as influenza shortly before their deaths, a finding of some interest considering the alleged capacity of viral infections to cause severe depression. Unfortunately, it is singularly difficult to prove a direct relationship between what is loosely called influenza, on the one hand, and affective disorder, on the other (71), and one can only speculate on whether being told about an upper respiratory infection before death persuaded the coroner to consider this to be an important factor causing depression and suicide.

Although Farberow and colleagues (8) reported an increase in patients with repiratory disease in their suicide series and Shapiro and Waltzer (69) found that patients with chronic obstructive pulmonary disease were overrepresented among their patients who made serious suicidal attempts, no other investigation has commented on this particular issue. Although some patients with severe respiratory distress might commit suicide, this is unlikely to be a mode of death occurring with significant frequency among patients with asthma and chronic bronchitis.

Musculoskeletal Disorders

One might expect an increase in suicide rates among patients suffering from severe arthritis, particularly because major depressive symptoms can be a complication of rheumatoid arthritis (72, 73). On the basis of Copeman's figures (74) for the prevalence of arthritic disease in Great Britain, the number of such cases in the 1000-suicide study should have been between 60 and 80 had they been based on radiological findings as Copeman's estimates were. The figure of 39 closely approximates the 43 derived from the General Practice morbidity study. Statistically, therefore, there was no increase in the frequency of musculoskeletal disorders in the EWTS investigation— which is not to say that *none* in that series became depressed and decided to bring to a premature end a prolonged period of pain and disability. The fact remains, however, that the majority of predominantly elderly patients with arthritis resign themselves with stoical fortitude to what many regard as one of the inevitable accompaniments of advancing years.

Apart from Dorpat and Ripley (3), who estimated the prevalence of rheumatoid arthritis among their 80 suicides to be 2 to 3 times greater than the expected number, most suicide studies have nothing to say on this topic.

Fifteen of the EWTS suicides were suffering from disabilities and pain following accidents and other injuries. None was paraplegic, but 2 cases had lost limbs through amputation. Shukla and colleagues (75) reported that 22% of amputees in India developed depressive psychoses and that 2 of 72 patients attempted to take their own lives. Wilcox and Stauffer (76) conducted a follow-up study of 420 patients with paraplegia or quadriplegia and estimated their suicide rate to be 15 times greater than that of the rest of the population in the U.S. Ten of Sainsbury's cases were said to have had deformities, but it is not clear precisely what this term means. Assuming for the moment that about one-half were handicapped by injury, the figure of 13/1000 is almost the same as the number in the EWTS study. Unfortunately, it is not possible to compare these findings with the general population prevalence of persons physically disabled by accident because these data are not immediately available.

Endocrine Disorders

In the EWTS series the frequency of patients with endocrine disease did not exceed chance expectation, but one important condition complicated by severe depression, Cushing's syndrome, was not recorded. Whereas depression and suicidal behavior often occur in patients with this condition, for obvious reasons, those who commit suicide before receiving treatment will not be included in most follow-up studies of patients who have been treated. Nonetheless, Williams (77) has written: "In the past death commonly resulted among patients with Cushing's Disease from infections . . . and suicide." Starr (78) found that severe depression developed in about one-quarter of 53 patients, 10% of whom made suicidal attempts. This was estimated to be 1000 times greater than the general population rate. The figures for moderate and severe depression and attempted suicide as given by Jeffcoate and co-workers (79) closely approximate those quoted by Starr, but other investigators (80–82) mention only suicidal ideation rather than actual attempts. Taft and associates (83), however, commenting on 16 deaths of 42 patients, considered that 3 of these were suicides. On the evidence from these studies one has to conclude that the risk of attempted and actual suicide by patients with Cushing's syndrome is a considerable one and more likely to happen if the patient becomes deeply depressed.

Although suicidal behavior is unusual among patients with thyrotoxicosis, two recent communications (84, 85) have reported an association between violent suicide and this disease. It was suggested that some abnormality of the hypothalamic-pituitary-thyroid axis was responsible for this phenomenon.

Although severe depression and suicidal attempts have been reported among patients with hyperparathyroidism, instances of suicide appear to be most unusual. The present author has personal knowledge of two patients who made suicidal attempts in a setting of depression but who recovered when their parathyroid tumors were removed.

Other Conditions

Twenty patients in the EWTS study were described as suffering from chronic ill health, a term, no doubt, which would include many of the other specified diseases in this investigation. In the absence of fuller details and any comparison group, it is not possible to say whether this number represents an excess or underestimate of patients with this kind of diagnosis among suicides.

Three other conditions with increased suicide rates should be mentioned: anorexia nervosa, Klinefelter's syndrome, and acute intermittent porphyria. All of these disorders are relatively uncommon, although the number of patients with anorexia nervosa is said to be increasing. Theander (86) considered the rate of suicide among anorexia nervosa patients to be about the same as that of female psychiatric patients but 20 times greater than the rest of the female population. Nielsen (87) found that the suicide rate among patients with Klinefelter's syndrome and other sex chromosome abnormalities to be higher than expected, and patients with acute intermittent porphyria may become depressed and suicidal (88).

Surgical Operations. Both the London and Seattle studies reported a high incidence of suicide victims who had recently undergone surgical operations. In the latter study the rate was estimated to be 3.5 times greater than expected. At least 5 (4.1%) of Stewart's cases and 4 (3%) of the Brisbane suicides had recently received surgical treatment. It is difficult to obtain accurate data on the frequency of major surgical operations carried out each year on members of the general population, but according to one report (89) the rate of surgical procedures/1000 patients would be about 37.3. From this number must be deducted operations carried out on children and what are usually termed minor operations, thus giving a final estimate of about 21.7/1000/year. None of the suicide studies in England and Wales has surgical operation figures as high as those from the Seattle investigation, as the rates vary from 1.5 to 1.8 times greater than the expected numbers, with Sainsbury's figures being almost the same as the general population rate. Precisely why there should be an excess of suicides following surgery is hard to say. Some of the patients would have been treated for cancer, which carries its own risk of suicide. Others probably were still suffering from some of the consequences of surgery or, possibly, were faced by further treatment which they could not bring themselves to consider after their earlier experiences. In both the London and EWTS studies some patients had taken their lives shortly before surgery could be carried out, an indication that for some patients such a prospect was more than they could contemplate.

SUMMARY AND CONCLUSIONS

The facts set out in the preceding pages have demonstrated clearly enough that a significant number of persons who commit suicide are suffering from one or more, often chronic, diseases; and that the older the victim is, the greater is the likelihood that physical illness will be at least one major factor determining this mode of death.

Not all conditions, however, are more prevalent among suicide cases than in other members of the community. As was expected, the evidence from this and other investigations has shown that patients with diseases of the central nervous system or suffering from cancer are more at risk for taking their own lives. Considering the potential that diseases of the brain and malignant neoplasms have for causing severe melancholia (70), these findings are not surprising.

Two other conditions—peptic ulceration and its treatment by partial gastrectomy, and genitourinary disease among elderly men—appear to constitute major hazards as far as accomplished suicide is concerned. With respect to gastric and duodenal ulcers, it is probable that alcoholism and consequential depression are significant causes of increased mortality from suicide among sufferers from these conditions. As for genitourinary diseases in the elderly male, apart from those who respond by becoming severely depressed, it is likely that some find the prospect of surgery and its aftermath so disagreeable that they choose to evade these contingencies by taking their own lives. It is important, therefore, that older patients with genitourinary symptoms or who have undergone surgery for their correction should be carefully followed up to ensure that there are no untoward sequelae, both physical and psychological.

Considering the effects that some endocrine diseases have on cerebral function, unexpectedly only a handful of these disorders was included in the EWTS study. Depression and suicidal attempts are not unusual accompaniments of Cushing disease, but today, fortunately, earlier diagnosis and more effective treatment may help to ensure that death by suicide is rare.

After adding up the numbers of victims in the EWTS series with cardiovascular, respiratory, and musculoskeletal diseases, the lack of any increase in the prevalence of these conditions compared with the rest of the population was noteworthy. Such diseases more often afflict older patients who also have the highest suicide rates. Some of these will be suffering from more than one illness and, possibly, it is the steady accumulation of impaired function that makes the depressed patient decide that he has had enough.

The conclusions to be drawn from these investigations are clear enough. It has been shown repeatedly that many cases of suicide have been in touch with psychiatrists or their general practitioners a relatively short time before their deaths. In such cases, presumably, the onset of melancholia was overlooked or the impact of physical illness—if present—was not fully appreciated. Hence, to forestall suicide by such patients, direct inquiries must be made about the patient's mood and possible suicidal intentions. It is sometimes feared that too direct questioning on this issue might precipitate the outcome one is most anxious to avoid. This is not the case, and many patients will welcome the opportunity to discuss their feelings which hitherto they have concealed almost as much from themselves as from their medical advisers.

The other conclusion to be understood is the need, as far as possible, to control distressing symptoms, particularly severe pain. Today, with so many analgesics at one's disposal, there should be no justification for any patient with, for example, terminal cancer not obtaining relief from unremitting pain when this develops. Too often effective analgesia with opiates is withheld lest the patient becomes dependent on the drug. The likelihood of this is small but hardly one of prime importance when dealing with the terminally ill.

Acknowledgment. I am indebted to Dr. Victor Siskind, Reader in Medical Statistics at the University of Queensland, for advice on statistical calculations.

References

1. Chynoweth R, Tonge JI, Armstrong J: Suicide in Brisbane—a retrospective psychosocial study. *Aust NZ J Psychiatry* 14:37–46, 1980.
2. Sainsbury P: *Suicide in London. An Ecological Study.* London, Chapman & Hall, 1955.
3. Dorpat TL, Ripley HS: A study of suicide in the Seattle area. *Compr Psychiatry* 1:349–359, 1960.
4. Stewart I: Suicide; the influence of organic disease. *Lancet* 2:919–920, 1960.
5. Myers DH, Neal CD: Suicide in psychiatric patients. *Br J Psychiatry* 133:38–44, 1978.
6. Barraclough BM: Suicide in the elderly. In Kay DWK, Walk A (eds): *Recent Developments in Psychogeriatrics.* Ashford, Kent, Headley Brothers, 1971, pp 87–98.
7. Stenbeck A, Achté KA, Rimón RN: Physical disease, hypochondria and alcohol addiction in suicides committed by mental hospital patients. *Br J Psychiatry* 111:933–937, 1965.
8. Farberow NL, Ganzler S, Cutter E, Reynolds D: An 8-year survey of hospital suicides. *Life Threatening Behav* 1:184–202, 1971.
9. Gatter K, Bowen D: A study of suicide autopsies 1957–1977. *Med Sci Law* 20:37–42, 1980.
10. *Morbidity Statistics from General Practice 1971–1972.* Studies in medical and population subjects, no. 36. London, Her Majesty's Stationery Office, 1979.

168 / *Suicide*

11. Derrick EH: Suicide and its prevention. *Med J Aust* 1:668–671, 1941.
12. Robins E, Murphy GE, Wilkinson RH, Gassner S, Kayes J: Some clinical considerations in the prevention of suicide based on a study of 134 successful suicides. *Am J Public Health* 49:888–899, 1959.
13. Seager CP, Flood RA: Suicide in Bristol. *Br J Psychiatry* 111:919–932, 1965.
14. Rorsman B: Suicide in psychiatric patients: a comparative study. *Soc Psychiatry* 8:55–66, 1973.
15. Edwards JE, Whitlock FA: Suicide and attempted suicide in Brisbane. *Med J Aust* 1:932–938, 989–995, 1968.
16. Jacobson S, Jacobson DM: Suicide in Brighton. *Br J Psychiatry* 121:369–378, 1972.
17. Anasstassopoulos G, Kokkini D: Suicidal attempts in psychomotor epilepsy. *Behav Neuropsychiatry* 1:11–16, 1969.
18. Hancock JC, Bevilacqua AR: Temporal lobe dysrhythmia and impulsive or suicidal behavior. *South Med J* 64:1189–1193, 1971.
19. Griesinger W: *Mental Pathology and Therapeutics* (translated by Robertson CL, Rutherford CL). London, New Sydenham Society, 1867.
20. Maudsley H: *Responsibility in Mental Disease.* London, Henry S King & Co, 1874.
21. Barraclough BM: Suicide and epilepsy. In Reynolds EH, Trimble MR (eds): *Epilepsy and Psychiatry.* Edinburgh, Churchill-Livingstone, 1981.
22. Matthews WS, Barabas G: Suicide and epilepsy: a review of the literature. *Psychosomatics* 22:515–524, 1981.
23. White SJ, McLean AEM, Howland C: Anticonvulsant drugs and cancer. (A cohort study in patients with severe epilepsy.) *Lancet* 2:458–461, 1979.
24. Zielinski JJ: Epilepsy and mortality rate and cause of death. *Epilepsia* 15:191–201, 1974.
25. Kahana E, Lebowitz W, Alter M: Cerebral multiple sclerosis. *Neurology (Minn)* 21:1179–1185, 1971.
26. Kellner CH, Davenport Y, Post RM, Ross RJ: Rapidly cycling bipolar disorder and multiple sclerosis. *Am J Psychiatry* 141:112–113, 1984.
27. Whitlock FA, Siskind M: Depression as a major symptom of multiple sclerosis. *J Neurol Neurosurg Psychiatry* 43:861–865, 1980.
28. Lishman WA: *Organic Psychiatry.* Oxford, Blackwell Scientific Publications, 1978.
29. Lewin W, Marshall TFdeC, Roberts AH: Long-term outcome after severe head injury. *Br Med J* 2:1533–1538, 1979.
30. Achté KA, Anttinen EE. Suizide bei Hirngeschadigten des Krieges in Finnland. *Fortschr Neurol Psychiatr* 31:645–667, 1963.
31. Vauhkonen K: Suicide among the male disabled with war injuries to the brain. *Acta Psychiatr Scand* (suppl 137), 90–91, 1959.
32. Maneros A, Philipp M: Zyklothymic und Hirnstamm. *Psychiatr Clin* 11:132–138, 1978.
33. Brewin M, Poskanzer DC, Rolland C, Miller H: Neurological disease in an English city. *Acta Neurol Scand* 42 (suppl 24), 1966.
34. Folstein MF, Maiberger R, McHugh PR: Mood disorder as a specific complication of stroke. *J Neurol Neurosurg Psychiatry* 40:1018–1020, 1977.
35. Storey PB: Psychiatric sequelae of subarachnoid haemorrhage. *Br J Psychiatry* 117:129–142, 1970.
36. Logue V, Durward M, Pratt RTC, Piercy M, Nixon WCB: Quality of survival after rupture of anterior cerebral aneurysm. *Br J Psychiatry* 114:137–160, 1968.
37. Huntington G: On chorea. *Med Surg Rep (Phila)* 26:317–321, 1872.
38. Folstein SE, Abbott MH, Chase GA, Jensen BA, Folstein MF: The association of affective disorder with Huntington's disease in a case series and in families. *Psychol Med* 13:537–542, 1983.
39. Oltman JE, Friedman S: Comments on Huntington's chorea. *Dis Nerv Syst* 22:313–319, 1961.
40. Chiu E, Alexander L: Causes of death in Huntington's disease. *Med J Aust* 1:153–154, 1982.
41. Reed TE, Chandler JH: Huntington's chorea in Michigan. I. Demography and genetics. *Am J Hum Genet* 10:201–225, 1958.

42. Oliver JE: Huntington's chorea in Northamptonshire. *Br J Psychiatry* 116:241–253, 1970.
43. Henry GW: Mental phenomena observed in cases of brain tumour. *Am J Psychiatry* 89:415–473, 1932.
44. Keschner M, Bender MB, Strauss I: Mental symptoms associated with brain tumour. *JAMA* 110:714–718, 1938.
45. Mindham RHS: Psychiatric symptoms in Parkinsonism. *J Neurol Neurosurg Psychiatry* 33:188–191, 1970.
46. Schneider E, Fischer PA, Jacobi P, Kolb R: Mortalität beim Parkinsonsyndrom und ihre Beeinflussung durch L-Dopa. *Fortschr Neurol Psychiatr* 49:187–192, 1981.
47. Parant V: Paralysis agitans: insanity associated with. In Tuke DH (ed): *Dictionary of Psychological medicine.* London, Churchill, 1892, pp 844–886.
48. Whitlock FA: Suicide, cancer and depression. *Br J Psychiatry* 132:269–274, 1978.
49. Fox BH, Stanek EJ, Boyd SC, Flannery JT: Suicide rates among cancer patients in Connecticut. *J Chronic Dis* 35:89–100, 1982.
50. Louhivuori KA, Hakama M: Risk of suicide among cancer patients. *Am J Epidemiol* 109:59–65, 1979.
51. Whitlock FA: Some psychiatric consequences of gastrectomy. *Br Med J* 1:1560–1564, 1961.
52. Krause V: Long-term results of medical and surgical treatment of peptic ulcer. *Acta Chir Scand* (suppl 310), 1963.
53. Westlund K: Mortality of peptic ulcer patients. *Acta Med Scand* (suppl 402), 1963.
54. Knop J, Fischer A: Duodenal ulcer, suicide, psychopathology and alcoholism. *Acta Psychiatr Scand* 63:346–355, 1981.
55. Ross AHMcL, Smith MA, Anderson JR, Small P: Late mortality after surgery for peptic ulcer. *N Engl J. Med* 307:519–522, 1982.
56. Hagnell O, Wretmark K: Peptic ulcer and alcoholism: a statistical study in frequency, behaviour, personality traits and family occurrence. *J Psychosom Res* 2:35–44, 1957.
57. Lereboullet J, Pluvinage R, Jungers P: Alcoholisme et gastrectomie. *Bull Soc Med Hôp Paris* 71:833–838, 1955.
58. Martimor E, Dereux JF, Nicholas-Charles P: Les donnés statistiques sur la frequence de gastrectomies chez les éthiliques. *Presse Méd* 64:1393–1394, 1956.
59. Navratil L, Wenger R: Alkoholismus und magengeschwür. *Münch Med Wochenschr* 97:1457–1459, 1955.
60. Soeder M: Trunksucht nach magenresektion. *Nervenarzt* 28:228–229, 1957.
61. Carney MWP, Sheffield BF: Crohn's disease: a psychosomatic illness? *Br J Psychiatry* 128:446–450, 1976.
62. Pons J: Sympathetic insanity. In Tuke DH (ed): *Dictionary of Psychological Medicine.* London, Churchill, 1892, p 1246.
63. Fawcett J: Suicidal depression and physical illness. *JAMA* 219:1303–1306, 1972.
64. Blandy J (ed): *Urology.* Oxford, Blackwell Scientific Publications, 1976, p 886.
65. Dunlop JL: Psychiatric aspects of urology. *Br J Psychiatry* 134:436–438, 1979.
66. Lowry MR: Frequency of depressive disorder in patients entering home dialysis. *J Nerv Ment Dis* 167:199–204, 1979.
67. Haenel T, Brunner F, Battegay R: Renal dialysis and suicide: occurrence in Switzerland and in Europe. *Compr Psychiatry* 21:140–145, 1980.
68. Abrams HS, Moore GL, Westervelt FB: Suicidal behavior in chronic dialysis patients. *Am J Psychiatry* 127:1199–1204, 1971.
69. Shapiro S, Waltzer H: Successful suicides and serious attempts in a general hospital over a 15-year period. *Gen Hosp Psychiatry* 2:118–126, 1980.
70. Whitlock GA: *Symptomatic Affective Disorder.* New York, Academic Press, 1982.
71. Sinaman K, Hillary I: Post-influenzal depression. *Br J Psychiatry* 138:131–133, 1981.
72. Labhardt F, Muller W: Psychosomatische aspekte rheumatischer in besondere weichteilrheumatische erkrankungen. *Schweitz Med Wochenschr* 106:1912–1917, 1976.
73. Editorial: Mental problems in rheumatoid arthritis. *Br Med J* 4:319, 1969.
74. Copeman WSC: *Textbook of the Rheumatic Diseases.* Edinburgh, E & S Livingstone, 1964.
75. Shukla GD, Sahu SC, Tripathi RP, Gupta DK: A psychiatric study of amputees. *Br J*

Psychiatry 141:50–53, 1982.
76. Wilcox E, Stauffer ES: Follow-up of 423 consecutive patients admitted to the spinal cord centre. *Paraplegia* 10:115–122, 1972.
77. Williams R: In Williams R (ed): *A Textbook of Endocrinology.* Philadelphia, WB Saunders, 1981, p 269.
78. Starr AM: Personality changes in Cushing's syndrome. *J Clin Endocrinol* 12:502–505, 1952.
79. Jeffcoate WJ, Silverstone KT, Edwards CRW, Besser GM: Psychiatric manifestations of Cushing's syndrome: response to lowering of plasma cortisol. *Q J Med* 48:465–472, 1979.
80. Rubin RT, Mandell AJ: Adrenocortical activity in psychological emotional states: a review. *Am J Psychiatry* 123:387–400, 1966.
81. Starkman MN, Schteingart DE: Cushing's syndrome: a prospective study. *Psychosom Med* 41:72–73, 1969.
82. Spillane JD: Nervous and mental disorders in Cushing's syndrome. *Brain* 74:72–98, 1951.
83. Taft P, Martin FIR, Mellick R: Cushing's syndrome: a review of the response to treatment in 42 patients. *Australas Ann Med* 4:295–303, 1970.
84. Linkowski P, Van Wettere JP, Kerkhof M, Brauman H, Mendlevicz J: Thyrotrophin response to thyrostimulin in affectively ill women: relationship to suicidal behaviour. *Br J Psychiatry* 143:401–405, 1983.
85. Drummond L, Lodrick M, Hallstrom C: Thyroid abnormalities and violent suicide. *Br J Psychiatry* 144:213, 1984.
86. Theander S: Anorexia nervosa: a psychiatric investigation of 94 female patients. *Acta Psychiatr Scand* (suppl 214), 1976.
87. Nielsen J: Klinefelter's syndrome and the XYY syndrome. *Acta Psychiatr Scand* (suppl 209), 1964.
88. Stein JA, Tschudy DP: Acute intermittent porphyria: a clinical and biochemical study of 46 patients. *Medicine* 49:1–16, 1970.
89. *Hospital Inpatient Enquiry 1978*, Series MB4 No 12. London, Her Majesty's Stationery Office, 1979.

12

The Physician's Role in Suicide Prevention

George E. Murphy, M.D.

Physicians have a unique role to play in suicide prevention. Self-destruction rarely occurs in the absence of clinical illness (98%) and particularly (over 90%) of psychiatric illness (1–5). The clinical conditions that predispose to suicide frequently occasion visits to physicians, mostly nonpsychiatrists. In fact, half or more of suicides have consulted a physician within a month or less of their death with complaints related to the psychiatric illness (1). When this level of attention is compared to the 3 to 6% of suicides who have had prior contact with a public agency whose mission is suicide prevention, it can be seen that the physician's office is the primary suicide prevention center.

It is not simply a matter of being clinically ill or even psychiatrically ill that predisposes a person to suicide. Certain psychiatric illnesses are intimately connected with this type of fatal outcome, while others are not. Affective disorders, in the depressed phase, have been found repeatedly to be most often present; proportions range from 30% (2) to 80% (3) in various studies. Alcoholism accounts for an additional 20 to 30% (1, 2, 4, 5). Together, these two common and readily recognizable psychiatric conditions are present in two-thirds or more of suicidal deaths. Smaller contributions are made by schizophrenia and by organic brain syndromes (dementia and delirium).

Antisocial personality and somatization disorder (Briquet's syndrome, hysteria) are infrequent contributors unless complicated by substance abuse. Anxiety disorders (phobic disorder, panic disorder, generalized anxiety disorder) have rarely been diagnosed. (When viewed from a cause of death perspective, however, suicide is not so rare an outcome for panic disorder and generalized anxiety disorder (6).) The manic or hypomanic state of bipolar affective disorder has not been reported once in over 720 cases where attention has been given to clinical diagnosis (1–5, 7). It behooves every physician to be familiar with the diagnoses of depressive disorder and alcoholism, since *clinical diagnosis is the key to effective treatment.* The *Diagnostic and Statistical Manual of Mental Disorders* criteria for the diagnosis of major depressive disorder are listed in Table 12.1. Those for alcohol abuse and alcohol addiction are listed in Chapter 6.

ERRORS OF OMISSION

Physicians fail to recognize and to deal with suicidal risk for a variety of reasons. The most prominent of these is simply missing the psychiatric diagnosis (8). Thirty

Table 12.1. DSM-III Criteria for the Diagnosis of Major Affective Disorder, Depressed*

A. Dysphoric mood or loss of interest or pleasure in all or almost all usual activities and pastimes
B. At least four of the following symptoms, each having been present nearly every day for at least 2 weeks:
   1. Poor appetite or significant weight loss, or increased appetite or significant weight gain
   2. Insomnia or hypersomnia
   3. Psychomotor agitation or retardation (not merely subjective)
   4. Loss of interest or pleasure in usual activities, or decrease in sexual drive not limited to a period when delusional or hallucinating.
   5. Loss of energy, fatigue
   6. Feelings of worthlessness, self-reproach, or excessive or inappropriate guilt
   7. Diminished ability to think or concentrate, slowed thinking, or indecisiveness
   8. Recurrent thoughts of death, suicidal ideation, wishes to be dead, or suicide attempt
C. Neither preoccupation with a mood-incongruent delusion or hallucination or bizarre behavior dominates the clinical picture when an affective syndrome is absent (symptoms in criterion A or B, above)

* From American Psychiatric Association: *Diagnostic and Statistical Manual of Mental Disorders*, ed 3. Washington, DC, American Psychiatric Association, 1980, pp 213–214.

years ago, so little could be done for the psychiatrically ill that psychiatric diagnosis seemed largely irrelevant. Treatment began to improve in the 1950s with the introduction of the major tranquilizers and antidepressants. However, the benefits were slow to be appreciated. The introduction of lithium carbonate therapy as an apparent specific therapy for mania made it meaningful to distinguish one form of psychotic behavior from another because of the striking clinical response of mania to this agent. The tardy acceptance by American psychiatry of the significance and value of systematic psychiatric diagnosis has resulted in graduating huge numbers of physicians into the practice of medicine who were never presented with practical and realistic knowledge in this domain.

The publication in 1972 of research diagnostic criteria for psychiatric diagnoses (9) brought together the work of a small but dedicated group of clinician-scholars to form the needed basis for systematic classification in American psychiatry. The third edition of *The Diagnostic and Statistical Manual of Mental Disorders* (DSM-III) of the American Psychiatric Association (10) in 1980 broadened these criteria somewhat for greater utility in clinical as opposed to research settings. DSM-III gave official sanction to systematic, criterion-based psychiatric diagnosis in the U.S. Both the research and the clinical diagnostic criteria had built on earlier natural history studies of psychiatric illnesses, having their roots in the European and British descriptive tradition. Among other advances, DSM-III does not assume etiology for most of the diagnostic categories. (DSM-II had assigned them indiscriminately to the category of "*reactions*.") The benefits of the recent changes in diagnostic style are to be seen in rapid growth and sophistication of systematic studies of treatment outcomes. Pharmaceutical firms have played a significant role in familiarizing physicians with the indications for use of their highly profitable products. Physicians graduating from medical school this year will have little excuse for unfamiliarity with the major psychiatric disorders or their current treatment. Many clinicians in practice have some catching up to do.

Symptoms versus Syndrome

Diagnosis is the key to appropriate treatment in all clinical medicine, and no less so in the recognition of suicidal risk. Missing the diagnosis is not solely a function of lack of familiarity with published diagnostic criteria. The right questions have to be asked. If they are not asked, they are unikely to be answered. Patients rarely present to the nonpsychiatric physician with a complaint of, "I'm depressed." They may complain of feeling nervous or upset and receive an anxiolytic. The patient who complains of loss of appetite or weight loss is likely to receive a gastrointestinal workup before the negative result forces the physician to take a more comprehensive clinical history. A complaint of fatigue may elicit hematological and thyroid studies. Any one of the common symptoms of depression should trigger systematic inquiry as to the presence or absence of the other symptoms comprising the syndrome.

Symptomatic treatment has a long and honorable history in medicine. But syndromes, groups of symptoms occurring together, give symptoms heightened meaning. When a physician first treats the patient's complaint of insomnia with a hypnotic, he or she may later treat the same patient's complaint of fatigue with thyroid supplement or a stimulant. Murphy (8) found the symptomatic treatment approach a common reason for overlooking the diagnosis of depression in a series of suicides. Often, the patient had been under treatment for another condition. The onset of depression has been insidious, or apparently so. By treating a series of symptoms in turn, the pattern was overlooked. *Failure to think syndromically results in missed diagnoses.*

Psychological Mindedness

Oddly, "psychological mindeness" can lead to missing a psychiatric diagnosis (8). The physician who knows his patient well may be aware of the presence of environmental stressors. He/she may assume that these account for the changed mood or psychological distress. The "explanation" thus derived is allowed to end the search for a more general cause of distress. To avoid this error it is well to keep in mind Fawcett's (11) trenchant aphorism, "The presence of a reason for depression does not constitute a good reason for ignoring its presence."

Failure to Ask

The most direct way to assess suicidal risk is to ask the patient whether he has been entertaining such thoughts. Patients will usually admit it if they are, but they do not volunteer the information. Failure to ask about suicidal thoughts is unfortunately frequent. In two separate studies of suicide, conducted 15 years apart Murphy (8) and Robins et al (12) found that only one of six physicians had known of the suicidal preoccupations of the patients who took their lives. This was true in spite of the fact that the information was readily available from others.

It is commonly thought that physicians avoid inquiring about the patient's suicidal ideas for fear of planting the thought in the patient's head. Such a fear has been widely (and wisely) discounted by experts in the field. An even less cogent reason is the fear of somehow embarrassing the patient. In the present writer's view, the question is most frequently avoided because of the physician's reluctance to hear unsettling news. Death is the physician's traditional enemy. Many find it difficult to deal with the idea that a patient would deliberately inflict on him/herself what we work so hard to postpone.

After clinical diagnosis, the next most important step in risk assessment is to ask about suicidal thoughts. The question need not be abrupt. Upon recognizing that the patient has been feeling unwell, a compassionate question is, "Have you sometimes thought life was not worth living?" Next, "Have you sometimes wished you were dead?" If the answer is yes, "Have you thought of doing anything about it?" Finally, "What have you thought of doing?" *The patient who has formulated a potentially lethal plan and secured the means for its execution is at high risk and should be hospitalized forthwith on a closed psychiatric unit for treatment.*

Playing the Odds

Undue reliance on commonly cited predictors of suicide may blunt the clinician's alertness to risk. A majority of suicides are males. The suicide rate is higher among the single, widowed, and divorced as compared to the married. Until recently, suicide was more common among those over the age of 40. While the statistics are correct, the guidance they offer is illusory. For example, although males are at greater risk for suicide than females, a majority of physician visits are by women. Furthermore, women are twice as likely as men to be clinically depressed. Thus, there may be nearly as many suicidal women as suicidal men in a general medical practice.

While the single, widowed, and divorced are at statistically higher risk, nearly three-fourths of adults in our population are married. As a consequence, most suicides occur among the married. Looking at a consecutive series of suicides from this viewpoint, it can be seen that if all males over the age of 40 who were single, widowed, or divorced had been prevented from taking their lives, the proportion of suicides so prevented would be less than 20% of the total (13). Demographics can, at best, alert one to special areas of high risk. They will not identify patients at low risk.

Undertreatment

Undertreatment also characterizes the population of suicides under medical care. Too often an anxiolytic has been prescribed instead of an antidepressant. If an antidepressant was prescribed, it was in an amount far below that customarily employed by psychiatrists (3, 8). To be sure, nonpsychiatric physicians deal with a different clinical population than psychiatrists do—one in which many respond to rather low doses of antidepressant medication. However, if the patient is not responding at a low dose, he or she should be treated more vigorously or referred to a psychiatrist for more aggressive intervention.

In addition to too little medication, retrospective studies of suicide show frequent omission of needed hospitalization (1, 7, 8). This need was not judged to have been present because of the fact that the patient took his or her own life. Rather, the usual indications for hospitalizations were considered—active suicidal ideation, depressive delusions, agitation, retardation, inability to fulfill one's customary role. It is not uncommon to encounter suicides with a history of electroconvulsive therapy (ECT) for an earlier episode of depression. Very rarely have suicides been so treated in the episode leading to their death. ECT has the potential for being a lifesaving procedure. The declining use of ECT in recent years has been paralleled by an increase in the suicide rate. *Severe depression, equivalent to melancholia, is a clear call for ECT.*

Hospital Discharge

Among persons ever hospitalized for psychiatric illness, the suicide rate is highest in the days and weeks following discharge (14). Current hospitalization costs make early discharge a desirable goal, all else being equal. Third-party payers press constantly for reduced hospital stays. Often patients are not kept in the hospital long enough to be fully stable. However, it is not simply a matter of sending patients home too soon.

Discharge from the hospital is commonly the beginning of a period of sharply curtailed physician support and surveillance. It is likely that the patient was seen by the physician almost daily while in the hospital. On discharge he or she may be given a follow-up appointment 2, 4, or even 6 weeks in the future. This may be experienced by the patient as abandonment. The mood fluctuations that frequently characterize the recovery phase of depression may be interpreted by the patient as relapse. In the absence of close contact with the physician, there is little opportunity to correct such misapprehensions. Despair may ensue, and then suicide. *Close follow-up in the immediate posthospital period is a sound precaution, with careful monitoring of suicidal thinking.*

ERROR OF COMMISSION

Along with undertreating (of the depression) goes overtreating (usually of symptoms). Too much of something is prescribed. In a study of suicides by overdose, Murphy (15) found that a lethal amount of a hypnotic had been prescribed in half of the cases within a week or less of the suicide. In some cases, the prescription had been given without a clinical history having been taken. Physicians are sometimes simply too compliant with their patients' requests for hypnotic medication. This study was conducted when barbiturates were still the predominant hypnotics in use. Today, a far less toxic benzodiazapine is likely to be prescribed. This change in prescribing practices is reflected in the structure of drug "mentions" of the Drug Abuse Warning Network (DAWN) (16). Secobarbital (Seconal) moved from fourth among mentions in 1974 to eleventh among mentions in 1982. Today, amitriptyline has fourth ranking, behind alcohol (in combination), heroin, and quinine (which is often used to "cut" illicit narcotics).

The practice by DAWN of listing specific compounds rather than classes of drugs obscures the probably larger role of antidepressants in overdose deaths. Many of the deaths by overdose may be accidental, but hardly those from antidepressants. The amount of antidepressant dispensed at a given time, both in newly acquired and in suicidally inclined patients, should be carefully considered. Even a week's supply, ingested as a bolus, may prove fatal. Frequent refills are an inconvenience both to the patient and the physician that must be weighed against the magnitude of the potential damage. Not only the pain of realizing that a lethal miscalculation has been made, but also a lawsuit for wrongful death may be avoided by closely supervised dispensing in high risk cases.

Murphy (8) found no evidence of stockpiling in anticipation of suicide in a series of overdose deaths. Half of the patients ingested the lethal prescription they had just received. The other half took a combination of things from the medicine cabinet. Stockpiling may, of course, occur, and there is little the physician can do to prevent a deliberate attempt to circumvent his therapeutic caution. The point is that sometimes physicians are insufficiently cautious.

FURTHER PRECAUTIONS

When suicidal risk is recognized, steps must be taken to protect the patient. If hospitalization is refused or postponed, a serious effort must be made to reduce the availability of lethal options. Instructing the family to remove all firearms from the premises ·is basic. An inventory of the medicine cabinet will likely reveal some unneeded risks. Propoxyphene is rarely the sole ingestant in overdose deaths. However, it receives remarkably frequent mention among drugs ingested with lethal outcome when a combination is employed. This drug should not be allowed to accumulate in the medicine cabinet.

It is virtually impossible to make a home completely suicide proof. If all ropes and belts are locked away, a wire coat hanger may still provide the suicidally motivated patient with a mode of exodus. Likewise, knives, broken glass, plastic bags, bathtubs, and electrical appliances have all be used with lethal effect. When the suicidal drive is strong, home is no place for the patient. Secure psychiatric hospitalization is essential.

Suicidal intent is not a long enduring state, and suicide is a rare occurrence. Thus, the reader may recognize having broken any number of the recommendations given above on various occasions without dire consequences. That is no guarantee that the same situation will prevail in the future. Suicide is irreversible. The steps to prevent it are uncertain. Recognition and treatment of the underlying psychiatric illness are basic. In addition, *the clinician will want to avoid facilitating a suicide by careless prescribing.*

"PREDICTING" SUICIDE: THE PROPERTIES OF A RARE EVENT

Over the years, the hope has persisted that a more accurate way would be found for identifying patients at high risk of suicide. Analog studies with suicide attempters have been undertaken with this hope in mind. However, the yield has ranged from confusing to nonexistent because of the fact that suicide attempt is fundamentally a different problem with a different population, and a different background from suicide (17, 18). What makes the problem of refining the identification of high risk patients so difficult is the fact that suicide is a rare phenomenon. It occurs at a rate of about 12.5/100,000 live persons/year in the United States. The statistical properties of rare events dictate that it will be extremely difficult, if not impossible, to identify those at risk with any degree of precision against the background of normality.

To be clinically useful, a test for a condition must have a high degree of *sensitivity*; that is, it must have the ability to detect positive cases among all cases tested. It must also have a high degree of *specificity*. That is, it must not misidentify as positive those cases that are, in fact, negative. A test that is 90% sensitive will identify 9 of 10 cases in which the condition is present. A test that is 99% specific will give a negative response in 99 of 100 unaffected cases.

For common conditions, such a test would be more than satisfactory, as, for example, in gallbladder disease. When the *base rate* of a phenomenon, the frequency of its occurrence in a population, is quite low, a test that is 99% specific (false positive rate 1%) will identify large numbers of patients falsely simply because there are large *numbers* of them evaluated. The magnitude of the effect on clinical prediction when the base rate is quite low may be difficult to conceptualize. It seems almost counter-intuitive.

What happens to clinical prediction in the face of very low base rates has been discussed lucidly by Galen and Gambino (19). To illustrate the problem, they cite actual experience in the detection of phenylketonuria (PKU). The incidence of this congenital metabolic disorder is between 5 and 10/100,000 live births. This is close enough to the annual incidence of suicide in the United States (around 12.5/100,000 living persons) to bring the point home. Setting the cutoff point of urine phenylalanine at 6 mg/dl, the test for PKU is 100% sensitive. That is, all cases are identified: none is missed. At that level, the specificity of the test is 99.95%. It is a remarkably accurate test. However, owing to the low base rate of the disorder, 83% of the babies identified as positive did not have PKU!

An 83% false positive rate in the face of 100% sensitivity and 99.95% specificity seems almost unbelievable. It results from the fact that every newborn is required to be screened for PKU. Thus, huge numbers of babies are screened while the number of actual cases of PKU is very small. With only one baby in 20,000 misclassified, the consequence was 83 false positives for every 17 cases of PKU actually found. Obviously, the false positive rate must be reduced. By choosing 20 mg/dl as the cutoff point, a specificity of 99.99% was achieved. This substantially reduced the number of false positives. However, the sensitivity of the test was inevitably reduced and more than 20% of PKU babies were missed. Reducing the false positive rate generally has the effect of increasing the false negative rate.

While this illustration emphasizes the impact of a low base rate on case finding, it is not altogether applicable to the problem of suicide. Unlike PKU screening, not every person in the population is screened for suicide risk. Only those coming to medical attention will be so examined. Since virtully all suicides are known to have been psychiatrically ill, a further enrichment strategy would be to examine patients admitted to a psychiatric hospital. There, the base rate might be orders of magnitude higher than in the general population.

Pursuing this strategy, Pokorny (20) studied 4800 patients consecutively admitted to Veterans' Administration psychiatric inpatient services. Items were extracted from their histories that had been found in earlier studies to have an increased correlation with suicide. When the patients were followed up 4 to 6 years later, 67 were found to have committed suicide. This represented a suicide rate of 279/100,000 persons/year, 12 times the expected rate for veterans and 23 times that of the general population.

Not surprisingly, no single feature distinguished the suicides from the nonsuicides. A computer program compiled factors made up of one or more characteristics that correlated more highly with suicide than with nonsuicide. Stepwise discriminant function analysis selected weighted combinations of variables that appeared to have an increased chance of predicting suicide. Having identified these correlates of suicide, the computer was then asked to go through the patient material case by case and to predict suicide or no suicide. The computer was allowed to assume equal frequencies of suicide and nonsuicide in the sample. Under this assumption it identified more than half of the suicides correctly. However, there were 1200 false positive predictions, one-fourth of the total sample! Seventy-four percent of the patients were classified correctly.

Then the computer was instructed as to the actual base rates of the two outcomes in the sample. This resulted in classifying 98.6% of cases correctly. Specificity was 99.99%. Yet, not a single suicide was predicted! Being apprised of the actual probabilities, the computer did the actuarially correct thing. It predicted no suicide in every case. It could have done the same thing without the patient data. The clinician who predicts "no suicide" in every case will have a similarly high rate of correct prediction, while the suicides will all be unanticipated.

Motto (21, 22) studied an even more enriched population consisting of 3006 persons admitted to a psychiatric inpatient unit *because of a depressive or suicidal state.* Since the study was prospective, a larger number of items of a psychosocial nature was recorded. A total of 2953 patients were followed up after 2 years and the suicides were identified. Rather than employ conventional clinical diagnosis, Motto postulated that, "certain kinds of people constitute clinical models in that they tend to respond to a given constellation of stresses in a similar way with regard to suicidal behavior." He then divided his population into an index sample and a replication sample. In this way, he could develop predictor models from his first sample and try them for predictive power in the second sample. From the constellations of characteristics and outcomes, Motto reported three "clinical models" derived from this data. One was a subjectively diagnosed group of alcohol abusers (diagnostic criteria unstated). Another was characterized as "males under forty," and the third as "stable with forced change." The predictive variables that he identified in his index samples performed expectedly less well on two of the three replication sets. Deterioration was not so striking for the "stable with forced change" model. The proportion of suicides and nonsuicides in the total sample that conformed to one or more of the "clinical models" was not stated. The highest sensitivity achieved in any index subsample was 93%, with an 82% specificity. In the validation set, the greatest sensitivity was 64% with 66% specificity. From what has been said earlier, it must be clear that these levels of sensitivity and specificity will not usefully serve to identify prospective suicides in a clinical population.

These studies illustrate the unlikelihood of one's ever being able to make accurate predictions of suicide in the population by statistical manipulation. This is not as unfortunate as it might seem, because there is little utility in knowing that a given person may some day destroy himself. The problem that confronts the clinician is what the likelihood is that the patient sitting before him may commit suicide *in the near future.* The decision is not an actuarial, but a clinical one. As with any clinical problem, the question is not what the outcome will be but what the clinician should do next. Should he observe further? Should he prescribe medication? Should he refer to someone more experienced in the specific problem presented? Should he hospitalize the patient? In order to make any of these decisions, he must first arrive at a decision as to what psychiatric illness, if any, is present. If a diagnosis having a substantial association with suicide is made, assessment of immediate risk must be undertaken. Ask the patient about suicidal ideation. Ask the family if there has been communication of suicidal thinking. The great rarity of suicide in the absence of *active* major psychiatric illness shows that identification and treatment of the underlying psychiatric illness are the most direct routes to suicide prevention. That is the physician's role in the prevention of suicide (23).

References

1. Robins E, Murphy GE, Wilkinson RH Jr, Gassner S, Kayes J: Some clinical considerations in the prevention of suicide based on a study of 134 successful suicides. *Am J Public Health* 49:888–889, 1959.
2. Dorpat TL, Ripley HS: A study of suicide in the Seattle area. *Compr Psychiatry* 1:349–359, 1960.
3. Barraclough B, Bunch J, Nelson B, Sainsbury P: A hundred cases of suicide: clinical aspects. *Br J Psychiatry* 125:355–373, 1974.
4. Beskow J: Suicide and mental disorder in Swedish men. *Acta Psychiatry Scand (Suppl)* 277:1–138, 1979.
5. Chynoweth R, Tonge JI, Armstrong J: Suicide in Brisbane—a retrospective psychosocial study. *Aust NZ J Psychiatry* 14:37–45, 1980.
6. Coryell W, Noyes R, Clancey J: Excess mortality in panic disorder. A comparison with primary unipolar depressions. *Arch Gen Psychiatry* 39:701–703, 1982.
7. Murphy GE, Armstrong JW Jr, Hermele SL, Fischer JR, Clendenin WW: Suicide and alcoholism: interpersonal loss confirmed as a predictor. *Arch Gen Psychiatry* 36:65–69, 1979.
8. Murphy GE: The physician's responsibility for suicide. II. Errors of omission. *Ann Intern Med* 82:305–309, 1975.

9. Feighner JP, Robins E, Guze SB, Woodruff RA, Winokur G, Munoz R: Diagnostic criteria for use in psychiatric research. *Arch Gen Psychiatry* 26:57–63, 1972.
10. American Psychiatric Association, Committee on Nomenclature and Statistics: *Diagnostic and Statistical Manual of Mental Disorders*, ed 3. Washington, DC, American Psychiatric Association, 1980.
11. Fawcett J: Suicidal depression and physical illness. *JAMA* 219:1303–1306, 1972.
12. Robins E, Gassner S, Kayes J, Wilkinson RH, Murphy GE: The communication of suicidal intent: a study of 134 consecutive cases of successful (completed) suicide. *Am J Psychiatry* 115:724–733, 1959.
13. Murphy GE: Clinical identification of suicidal risk. *Arch Gen Psychiatry* 27:356–359, 1972.
14. Temoche A, Pugh RF, MacMahon B: Suicide rates among current and former mental institution patients. *J Nerv Ment Dis* 138:124–130, 1964.
15. Murphy GE: The physician's responsibility for suicide. I. An error of commission. *Ann Intern Med* 82:301–304, 1975.
16. National Institute on Drug Statistical Series. Annual Data, 1982. Data from the Drug Abuse Warning Network (DAWN). Series I, no. 2. Washington, DC, United States Department of Health and Human Services, 1983.
17. McCulloch JW: Social prognosis of an Edinburgh clientele. In Waldenström J, Larsson T, and Ljungstedt N (eds): *Suicide and Attempted Suicide.* Stockholm, Nordiska Bokhandels Forlag, 1972.
18. Kreitman N: *Parasuicide.* New York, John Wiley & Sons, 1977.
19. Galen RS, Gambino SR: *Beyond Normality. The Predictive Value and Efficiency of Medical Diagnoses.* New York, John Wiley & Sons, 1975, pp 123–125.
20. Pokorny AD: Prediction of suicide in psychiatric patients. *Arch Gen Psychiatry* 40:249–257, 1983.
21. Motto JA: The psychopathology of suicide: a clinical model approach. *Am J Psychiatry* 136:516–520, 1979.
22. Motto JA: Suicide risk factors in alcohol abuse. *Suicide Life Threat Behav* 10:230–238, 1980.
23. Murphy GE: The prediction of suicide: why is it so difficult? *Am J Psychother* 38:341–349, 1984.

13

The Clinical Assessment and Management of the Suicidal Patient

Norman Kreitman, M.D., F.R.C.P., F.R.C.Psych.

While the general physician expects to witness death fairly frequently in the course of his working day, such encounters are relatively infrequent for the psychiatrist. The only form of dying unique to his specialty is suicide, which is a rare phenomenon. Yet paradoxically it attracts more widespread interest from the larger society than any other mode of death. Suicide has always had a very special religious and legal significance, and indeed one of the most illuminating characteristics of a culture is how it accommodates self-destruction by its citizens. Creative writers have dealt with the theme since earliest times, and more recently a large body of comment and research has accumulated. When Emile Durkheim's *La Suicide* (1) first appeared in 1898 it was able, even at that time, to draw on over a century of sporadic scientific research (to say nothing of earlier speculative writings), while since the turn of the century behavioral scientists of all complexions have continued to pursue the theme with great vigor. The literature today is massive.

In this chapter an attempt will be made to summarize some of the pointers to the risk of suicide as it confronts the clinician. It is argued that the assessment of suicidal risk should be built up in layers, so to speak. The first level comprises general considerations such as might be derived from knowledge of the patient's location in the larger social unit, such as his social class or sex role. The second stage is based on the further consideration of possible pointers to suicide within the diagnostic or behavioral subgroup of which the patient is a member. Finally, attention is given to the individual features of the patient and his immediate social context. The constraints of space will in general mean focusing on the enumeration of prognostic features rather than exploring their dynamics in any depth; further, only the more important points can be considered, and the reader is referred to the more specialized chapters for further detail. Only after an assessment of risk has been more or less completed can appropriate steps then be taken for management and therapy. These stages will provide the framework of this chapter.

SOURCES OF DATA

To review the clinical presentation and management of the suicidal patient it is necessary to draw on three diverse sources of information. The first is the epidemiological and sociological research tradition already mentioned, using the analysis of variations in suicide rates between communities or between subgroups within single societies. Interestingly, such studies have also been found to translate into practice with a directness rare in other branches of psychiatric epidemiology. The psychiatrist who aspires to a competence in matters of suicide must familiarize himself with at least the basic epidemiology of the topic.

A second source of information is the corpus of clinical research utilizing follow-up studies. These permit an estimate to be made of the eventual risk of death by suicide within certain clinically defined groups. They are necessarily constrained by the limited character of the samples which have usually been available, and for the most part work of this kind is based on the more severely ill, as represented, for example, by inpatient cohorts. Useful summaries of such research have been presented by Pokorny (2) and by Guze and Robins (3), and an outpatient series has been investigated by Rorsman (4).

Complimentary to this approach is the analysis of series of suicides reviewed by clinicians, ideally using a random sample intensively studied, using documentary evidence and interview data from the deceased's family and other contacts. Such projects are difficult and expensive to mount, and few meet adequate standards (5–8). More limited inquiries can be carried through by concentrating on only those suicides who are known to have had a prior psychiatric contact (9–11). Investigations of this kind have certain limitations but may be particularly useful to clinicians since they help to suggest distinguishing features of patients who have gone on to suicide.

The third source of information is simply clinical expertise. Often what is of immediate clinical significance is the least extensively researched. Informal observation has to provide guidance until more secure information becomes available.

THE ASSESSMENT OF SUICIDAL RISK

The psychiatrist may encounter the potentially suicidal patient either in the course of routine clinical work or through involvement with patients who come to attention specifically because of acts of self-aggression. In either context the first set of evaluative criteria to be applied are nonspecific in the sense that they appear to hold good across all diagnostic categories and presentations; exceptions will be noted below.

General Predictors and Other Variables

1. Perhaps the most robust general finding to emerge is that *males* are at greater risk of suicide than females, though it is evident that the gap is rapidly closing.

2. In general those in the *second half of life* are at greater risk than younger patients, but the effects of age are a little different in the two sexes. Among men the rates increase more or less linearly with age, while among women the peak rates occur between 50 and 60 and thereafter decline. Over the last decade many western nations have reported a shift in the age-specific rates for both sexes, with a decrease in the rates for the elderly and an increase in the rates for the young. Nevertheless, the graph still shows a climb upward with increasing age, even if this is not as steep as was formerly the case.

3. *Social isolation* is one of the most extensively explored variables in suicide research. Epidemiological studies, however, have been obliged to use rather crude indicators of social isolation. These have been informative, but it is clear that what matters is psychological rather than geographical or physical isolation. It does not seem important for predictive purposes whether the isolation is a consequence of the individual's own actions, as, for example, following migration, or whether it is produced by events outside the individual's control, such as the death of a spouse.

4. *Marital status* has detailed implications. In both sexes the divorced have the highest suicide rates (especially after controlling for age). The basis for the association is complex. Marital breakdown may, of course, reflect psychopathology in the divorced individual, but in addition those who are divorced at time of death may represent a subgroup of divorced individuals who failed to remarry. It is also uncertain whether the high risk associated with divorce will persist as its social significance is changing so rapidly.

Among men the widowed have a raised risk of suicide. Widowhood has a less tangible effect among women, possibly because the latter are more able to sustain a home and a network of relationships. There is also evidence that among women being childless is an important predictor, whether or not the woman is a widow or married.

The state of being single, i.e., never having married, comes next in the ranking of risk factors, with married individuals last. It must be appreciated that marital status may also be a reflection of the age, sex, and social isolation variables already considered.

5. The presence of *physical illness* may also heighten suicidal risk. Some disorders, such as peptic ulceration, may conceivably reflect a chronic state of tension. More obviously, such conditions as arthritis in the elderly may be important both through being a chronically painful condition conducive to depression and also by constraining the social mobility of the individual so as to heighten isolation. Follow-up studies of groups of patients defined only by their particular physical disorder have yielded little in the way of an excess suicide rate, but physical disability certainly appears to potentiate the risk of those who are vulnerable for other reasons, as by virtue of an associated psychiatric disorder.

6. A former history of *self-damaging acts* predicts a higher rate of subsequent suicide than would be found among those who have no such history. This relationship can be demonstrated epidemiologically and is independent of specific diagnoses. The predictive significance of parasuicide is considered more fully below.

These general predictive factors can be amplified or modified according to the particular feature of subgroups of patients, in particular their diagnostic categories.

Suicide within Specified Groups

Affective Disorder

No study of a series of suicides has failed to demonstrate the major contribution made by affective disorders. Similarly, follow-up studies of depressive illness demonstrate that about 15% of patients with depressive illness, diagnosed according to standardized criteria such as the *Diagnostic and Statistical Manual of Mental Disorders* (12) or the Research Diagnostic Criteria (13) will eventually die by suicide (2). It seems that patients with affective disorder who proceed to suicide do so fairly early in their clinical career, often within the first year or two of clinical contact; thereafter suicides occur at a steady but lower rate. All the same, the alarming 15% figure, often quoted, overstresses short term risk since it refers to the group followed through their lives and hence spanning decades after the point of initial clinical contact. Moreover, it includes suicides in the setting of depressed episodes subsequent to the one which the clinician may initially encounter. The maximal risk of suicide appears to be toward the end of a depressive episode. Early commentators ascribed this to a lifting of psychomotor retardation occurring in a suicidal patient before improvement in mood, so that the patient was then able to put into operation impulses which he could not carry through earlier in his illness. This view is not well supported by the evidence. An alternative explanation is that the prospect of or actual termination of care may itself be traumatic, especially as the resolution of a depressive episode commonly takes much longer than the clinician or indeed the patient recognizes at the time. The conclusion is that contact should be maintained with depressed patients for a period well beyond the apparent resolution of their abnormal mood.

Many studies have looked at the endogenous/reactive dichotomy as a possible predictor for later suicide and have failed to demonstrate any difference. It is the intensity of the mood change which is important rather than the syndrome within which it occurs. Similarly, much effort has been expended in attempts to find ancillary predictive symptoms. Insomnia, impaired memory, and self-neglect have all been cited (14); so too has hopelessness concerning the future, a feature currently attracting much interest as a possible predictor of special importance (see below). In general, however, the quest for predictive symptoms has not been very successful, given the very large number that have been investigated. The nonspecific social variables cited above are of greater importance than the clinical details in the prediction of suicide, even within the depressive group.

Last, it must be remembered that sustained depression may occur in other psychiatric disorders. When it does so it is likely that the suicide risk is enhanced.

Alcoholism

Again the lifetime risk of suicide is commonly quoted at about 15%, but the usefulness of this estimate is rather less than for affective disorders since the diagnostic criteria employed have been considerably vaguer. In contrast to affective illness, it has been proposed that suicide in alcoholics tends to occur relatively later in the course of the disorder. It is known, for example, that suicide rates in a community tend to correlate more highly with cirrhosis rates than with rates for the treatment of clinical alcoholism.

A feature of suicide in this group is the recent history of loss by separation from a spouse or death of a parent (15). It does not seem to be relevant whether the isolation has been brought about by the patient's own actions or by fate. Insofar as the loss may be attributable to the deterioration in the patient's own drinking, it is possible that this variable is really reflecting clinical deterioration rather than isolation per se. Whatever the mechanism, a weakening of social ties by an individual who may already feel gloomy and inadequate might heighten his sense of despair and lead to suicide.

Alcoholics who kill themselves invariably do so during a phase when they are drinking heavily rather than during a remission. What is still unclear and in need of further research is the role of the alcohol dependence syndrome per se, of depression secondary to heavy drinking, of the associated social disruption, and of the possible role of personality disorder. Each should be separately considered when forming a clinical judgment.

Alcohol and Depression Together

It follows from what has already been stated that the concordance of clinical alcoholism plus severe depressive symptoms may be particularly dangerous. This would indeed appear to be the case. In cultures where drinking is common, a syndrome has been described in which an event, commonly the death of a parent befalling an unmarried son, triggers a pathological grief reaction; the mood change is then complicated by heavy drinking, often occurring for the first time in the individual's life. Suicide then follows. This pattern has been reported in up to a third of all suicides occurring in a consecutive series (16).

Schizophrenia

Recent work suggests that the eventual suicidal outcome of schizophrenics, traditionally cited at about 10%, has perhaps been underestimated. The potential suicide is particularly difficult to identify in this group; indeed apart from the greater susceptibility of males, the other "nonspecific" predictors do not appear to operate (17). There is little agreement as to which symptoms, if any, might indicate the patient most at risk. It is generally assumed that suicidal deaths occur in the framework of a delusional structure, but as these may develop or change rapidly the information is of little predictive value. There does not appear to be any evidence for the view that suicide usually occurs in schizophrenics in response to hallucinatory commands. On balance the likelihood of suicide among schizophrenics is better judged from the individual features mentioned in the next section rather than by review of the standard symptoms.

Personality Disorders and Neuroses

The point has been made that reactive depression, sometimes called depressive neurosis, does not carry a lower risk for eventual suicide than other types of affective disorder. The likelihood of suicide in connection with other neuroses is much lower, and for that reason it is difficult to assess accurately. Personality disorder, most commonly in the form of sociopathy, is certainly demonstrable in studies of suicides, but there are no worthwhile estimates of the likelihood of psychopaths dying by suicide since uncomplicated forms of abnormal personality, without neuroses or drug addiction, are relatively uncommon and difficult to follow up systematically.

Drug Addiction

This group, like the schizophrenics, is also difficult to assess in terms of the "general" criteria outlined above. It does indeed seem to hold that suicide among addicts is particularly a risk of males. It is also obvious that the suicidal deaths of drug addicts, when they can be clearly distinguished from deaths by misadventure, as from abusing drugs of ill specified strength, tend to occur in young people since addictions are much less common in the second half of life. There is sufficient evidence to show that drug addicts do indeed have an excess suicide mortality in comparison to the general population, but the extreme difficulties of systematic follow-up preclude any more precise statement. Miles (18) speculates that drug abuse may be the most important single factor in the increasing rates of suicide among youth in the United States.

Other Groups

It seems improbable that there is any diagnosable psychiatric condition which does not to some degree carry a heightened risk of suicide. The most notable have already been indicated. The question remains as to whether suicide ever occurs in individuals who are free of psychiatric disability.

One type of patient who is very difficult to treat is the somewhat isolated, intelligent youth whose integration with his peers is less than might ideally be wished but who could not be given a formal diagnosis according to any existing scheme. He presents to the psychiatrist not with a complaint or symptom but with questions about the ultimate meaning of life. Preoccupation with existential problems of this kind are common enough in the young, and most young people either grow used to their ignorance or find an acceptable answer. The kind of individual being described, however, will often indicate quite clearly that he anticipates finding no such outcome, and that he envisages suicide as the likely termination of his quest, though possibly not for some years. Such cases are rare and they do not figure in the classical studies of series of suicidal deaths. Nevertheless, the pattern appears to be sufficiently well established to be mentioned here.

It would be prudent to refrain from speculating as to what might have been the case in former times or what pertains nowadays in exotic cultures. Similarly, special circumstances operate within closed institutions such as prisons, or in organizations such as the military, especially in wartime. However, it seems that suicide does not occur among individuals with no psychiatric disability in western society and under normal peacetime conditions; the qualifications should be noted.

PARASUICIDE

This term was introduced to replace the misleading phrase "attempted suicide," since most patients so designated are not attempting to kill themselves. The epidemiology of parasuicide is quite distinct from that of suicide, and the clinical issues that arise in assessing and managing the parasuicidal patient are also different. To regard the patient simply as a failed suicide would gravely fail to meet clinical requirements. Nevertheless, the group of parasuicidal patients contains a small proportion who either at the time or subsequently are motivated by death-directed wishes. Most follow-up studies report a subsequent suicide rate of approximately 1 to 2%/ annum, continuing over at least 10 years (19). Of all clinically defined patient groups, parasuicides carry the highest risk for subsequent suicide.

The prediction of suicide following parasuicide has received much attention. Some decades ago Tuckman and Youngman (20, 21) proposed that the more closely a parasuicide approximated to the epidemiological profile of suicide the greater the risk of subsequent death from that cause. Their own data were somewhat limited, but their conclusions have been supported by independent research. Thus, for example, males have been found to have appreciably higher risk than females, and those in the older age group have higher risk than younger patients. Combining these characteristics thus enables one to distinguish subgroups with very differing risks. One follow-up study reported a rate of suicide of 8% over 2 years in men aged above 55 compared to a rate of 0.4% for women aged 15 to 34 years over the same period, i.e., a relative risk of 20 (22).

Presumably the episode serves to mark an individual in whom there are few inhibitions against self-aggression and hence liable to act on any suicidal impulses that might subsequently occur. It is also known that parasuicides who proceed to suicide have commonly accrued a number of parasuicidal episodes by the time of their death, though only occasionally do these follow a clear-cut progression of increasing severity. (It is worth noting, however, that those variables which predict to a repetition of *parasuicide* are not necessarily good predictors of ultimate suicide (23).)

The contribution of psychiatric diagnosis to prediction *within* the group of parasuicides is uncertain. Among those who subsequently die by suicide a diagnosis of personality disorder (at the time of the parasuicide) is particularly common, at least among males, and is often complicated by alcohol or drug abuse. The absence of depression from the list of predictive factors is interesting. Presumably patients who are depressed at the time of their parasuicidal episode and who are recognized as such are then taken into treatment, whereupon many will respond to antidepressant therapies. This is much less likely to be true for those diagnosed as alcoholics or as having personality disorders.

INDIVIDUAL FEATURES

The main risk factors to be borne in mind when assessing the possibility of suicide have now been listed, but many of these, such as demographic characteristics, are of a very general character and, though important, are scarcely sensitive enough to assist in identifying closely which individuals may be at particular hazard. Moreover, many of the features already discussed are established as predictors of suicide in the long term rather than the near future, whereas a clinician of course needs to address the immediate situation with more urgency than the distant future.

The finer grading of immediate or short term risk requires sensitive clinical assessment. Some of the main considerations are as follows:

1. Arguably the single most important clinical pointer is whether the patient is actively entertaining suicidal intention at the time of examination. It will be obvious that this question should be explored if the patient has presented as, say, a parasuicide but rather less so if he or she is seen as a routine, ambulatory referral with a complaint of inability to concentrate or loss of weight. The question should always be raised if there is the slightest suspicion in a clinician's mind. Fears that ventilating the subject may make suicide more likely are totally misplaced, while failure to inquire may lead to missing a patient at high risk. Though "seriousness of intention" is better established as a long range than a short term predictor (24), common sense alone would underline its significance, especially in the context of a parasuicidal act or a depressive illness.

Some patients will deny suicidal intention, but other features may make the clinician suspicious nevertheless. Denial here needs to be evaluated in the same way as any other item of information. It is worth mentioning that the patient who has just recovered from a highly dangerous parasuicide may indeed be telling the truth if he says he now has no suicidal intention, since there is often a powerful cathectic effect associated with self-damage. The correlation, incidentally, between the degree of physical damage and suicidal intent in parasuicide, though statistically significant, is too low to be of much use in a practical context.

2. Intensity of depressive affect is another major consideration. More specifically it appears that the component of the depressive syndrome which is of particular importance in the prediction of suicide is hopelessness or pessimism about the future (25, 26). Among parasuicides the hopelessness component of depression correlates more highly with suicidal intent than does mood change per se. This finding has not yet been verified for completed suicides, but it is likely to be substantiated.

3. There is a belief among experienced clinicians that patients whose suicidal ideas involve notions of reunions with a dead parent or spouse may be at particular hazard. This hypothesis has a certain plausibility.

4. The significance to be attached to a family history of suicide is somewhat uncertain; again, it might be important here to distinguish between the place that such a history has in the prediction of repeated parasuicide as contrasted to completed suicide (27). At one time investigators were sufficiently impressed with a familial clustering of suicide to speculate that it might have a specific genetic determinant. Opinion now would ascribe the clustering to the genetics of affective disorder and possibly of alcoholism, to which may be added the effect of role models and the force of example. It is certainly not established that suicide segregates in families after due allowance has been made for the transmission of psychiatric disorder per se. All the same a positive family history is a useful, if minor, predictive factor.

5. Last, it is worth mentioning that, although a patient at the moment of examination may show little in the way of marked depression or suicidal intent, a history of a recent phase during which these have been manifest, and of brittleness of mood,

should be noted. There is, for example, a subgroup of manic-depressive patients whose mood swings may develop very suddenly and who may be seriously suicidal in their depressed phases. Likewise there are certain kinds of personality disorder in which a salient characteristic is a propensity to intense though transitory depressive swings. Such patients are, of course, at risk even if on the day of examination there is little depression to elicit.

6. It has already been stressed that the social and interpersonal context of the patient is of major importance. Isolation in the objective sense is all too common among the elderly and the infirm (and the rate of suicide is demonstrably higher in single-person households). However, living alone does not necessarily reflect psychological isolation if the person is in regular and intimate contact with family and neighbors. Conversely, subjective isolation or loneliness may be felt by those living with others; it may either precede or follow the onset of illness. Hostile relationships, as in a long standing marital conflict, should also be noted because they may reflect an intense and hence sustaining involvement with others, but might also mean that the patient lacks appropriate support in times of crisis. The assistance of a social worker may be invaluable in dissecting out the subjective and objective components of the patient's environment and in reaching a just evaluation of the circumstances.

DISPOSITION AND GENERAL MANAGEMENT

Inpatient Care

The acutely suicidal patient is a psychiatric emergency and is preferably treated as an inpatient. Most suicidal patients are frightened of their own wishes and would like to feel differently and be relieved of the background of misery from which their intentions spring. It is nearly always possible to form a therapeutic alliance with the patient even if this is based on guilt at, for example, leaving behind dependent children or others who would grieve. Those patients least open to persuasion in this way are those with psychotic delusions or those in whom the depth of depression is such that they cannot credit any relief as possible. Fortunately their numbers are small. Nevertheless, they raise the question of the use of commitment procedures. In all legal systems a serious risk of suicide is a recognized basis for compulsion, which should be used if there is no alternative.

The management of suicidal patients in a psychiatric ward has changed considerably over the past few decades. At one time elaborate "suicide caution" routines were maintained whereby nursing staff kept the patient under close observation, usually on a one-to-one basis, and signed a card to say that they had been informed of the danger to the patient when they came on duty and that they had in turn relayed this information to their successors. The view nowadays is that such close watch is counterproductive; it is oppressive and induces restlessness and frustration in the patient to a greater degree than it reduces the opportunity for suicidal action. One exception to this generalization is when the patient herself requests the reassurance of having a staff member constantly and exclusively available. If staff are deployed in this way it should be as a short term arrangement from which the patient should be weaned as soon as possible. But the alternative to the "suicide caution" routine is not to take no particular steps but to have all nursing staff carefully appraised of the patient's clinical state. They should maintain continuous but unobtrusive observation and be particularly aware of the patient's need for assurance and support and of changes, for better or worse, in the patient's state. This in turn implies free and virtually trusting relationships between all members of the ward team.

It is also essential that the ward strategy should be clear and understood by all. If staff, particularly junior staff, are aware of exactly what procedures are required of them and that they will be fully supported by their senior colleagues in the event of misadventure provided agreed plans are carried out, their own anxiety will be much alleviated with consequent benefit to the patient. More generally it seems that a suicide is particularly apt to occur on a ward where there is confusion concerning responsibility, the roles of the various staff members, and the objectives which the ward is trying to attain.

The furbishings of the ward should be governed by common sense as well as esthetics. Ground floor accommodation is preferable; alternatively, windows should be so designed as to open only partially. Protuberances to which cords might be attached should be eliminated. Ward toilets should be designed as a compromise between privacy and the need for access in an emergency. Male patients judged at risk should be encouraged to use electric razors rather than safety razors. On the other hand, there is no reason why normal cutlery should not be used at mealtimes. The need for nursing staff to be aware of movement in the ward is particularly important and is much facilitated by a ward layout in which the senior nurse can observe the whole ward from the central nursing station.

Some of these points can be illustrated by considering briefly what is known of suicide occurring in inpatients, for whatever system is adopted such cases, tragically, will continue to occur. First, it seems that inpatient suicide is a particular hazard with newly opened institutions or where an existing hospital has been subject to a major reorganization. Presumably the common feature here is staff uncertainty concerning their role, with the subtle transmission of this anxiety to the patients. Second, it is well documented that inpatient suicides tend to occur in clusters or epidemics. The mechanism is uncertain. Case-to-case imitation is one possibility; it is certainly an aspect of the more general epidemiology of suicide which is receiving increasing attention. But it is also possible that the stressors attributable to the environment, such as staff anxiety as already mentioned, which contribute to the first suicide may continue to be active for some time, resulting in a series of further deaths. Third, it is evident that the method used will depend upon availability, hence the comments concerning the design and furbishing of the ward. At the same time it is important to recall that approximately half the suicides occurring among inpatients in psychiatric institutions take place while the patient is temporarily outside the hospital, as on weekend leave. The proportion is strikingly high and may be due to various factors. Among these could be included a wish by the patient to spare the staff from being directly implicated in their death, a greater access to methods of dying while outside the institution, and conceivably the presence of family members or others toward whom the suicide wishes specifically to direct his hostility. Fourth, efforts have been made to characterize the individual who while in hospital is particularly at risk. Most of these studies merely reiterate what has already been sketched concerning the high risk patient, but two further observations have been made. One is that the elderly seem to figure rarely in inpatient suicide statistics, and it is supposed the social isolation which is so important a factor in the suicide of the aged in the population is not operative within the institutional setting. The second point is that the individual destined to become an inpatient suicide often has a long story of abrasive relationships with the staff of the institution. Many authors comment that these patients are recognized early as "difficult"; they appear to seek confrontation, to ignore simple requests to assist in the smooth running of the ward, and gradually alienate the sympathy of all those around them. Such patients are, of course, very taxing, and staff can do little more than remind themselves of the importance of analyzing provocative behavior rather than simply responding to it.

Outpatient Care

The acutely suicidal patient being treated as an inpatient is being contained in the safest environment it is possible to devise. In some ways a more difficult problem is the decision as to whom to treat on an outpatient or ambulatory basis, and the knowledge that doing so inevitably entails some risk. Four points are relevant in making the decision.

First, the absolute risk of suicide, as judged by all of the criteria already reviewed, should be assessed as comparatively modest.

Second, the patient should enjoy the close support of his family and friends. Such support would itself mitigate the risk of suicide provided that the family is willing and able to provide continuing support for the patient. It is entirely reasonable to appraise the relatives, if they do not already know, that some risk of suicide exists, though often they will be only too keenly aware of this. On the other hand, it is most unjust to make relatives feel in any sense that they are the people primarily responsible for preventing a suicidal outcome. The physician must make it quite clear to the family that *he* is assuming the burden of decision as to where the patient is best managed.

Third, the patient's own wishes should as always be elicited and seriously considered. The points at issue would include not only the patient's preference for the setting in which he would wish his illness or problems to be treated but also specific questions of the management of suicidal impulses, such as the patient's confidence in controlling them, seeking help in a crisis, etc.

Last, outpatient care would be more appropriate, at least as an initial measure, for those whose disorders might be expected to respond fairly promptly to therapy.

Analogous problems arise with the decision about when to transfer a patient from inpatient to outpatient care. The residual risk of suicide will have to be balanced against the substantial gains from the reintegration of the patient in his normal routine and living group and of prolonging hospital stay no longer than is absolutely necessary. Any patient who at any time has been suicidal, particularly in association with a depressive episode, must always be assured of a line of support in the future. Outpatient appointments should be regular, and spaced at increasing intervals toward the end of therapy. The patient should be told that he or she may always make contact at any time should he/she wish. Many patients report that the knowledge that they can secure help often obviates the need for them to do so.

The clinician will have to face a further decision concerning the actual point of discharge from care. Often he will refer the patient back to a primary care physician or to some form of supporting service. When this occurs it is equally important for the new supporters themselves to be offered support either during a planned consultation or by an open invitation to request emergency guidance if required. The patient's spouse is often overlooked in this context, though he or she is possibly the most important of all the "caretakers" with whom the patient will come into contact.

GENERAL PRINCIPLES OF MANAGEMENT

The therapy and general management of the suicidal patient should be guided by two cardinal considerations. The first is whether the patient is receiving adequate treatment for the disorder which would have been diagnosed even in the absence of his suicidal ideas or acts. Specific therapies are most likely to be required if the patient is considered to be suffering from an affective disorder, the alcohol dependence syndrome, or schizophrenia. In the first of these it is worth stressing that the patient who is severely depressed and suicidal is in a state of great psychological pain. This implies that therapies should be used which are as rapid in their effects as possible, and in particular that electroconvulsive treatments (ECT) should not be withheld in order to experiment with antidepressant drugs. Indeed, the more severely depressed the patient, the more dramatic his response to ECT is likely to be. Once mood has been normalized subsequent management will, of course, proceed upon whatever lines the clinician habitually adopts. The value of ECT for depressive states associated with other disorders such as schizophrenia is very much less clear-cut. While there is evidence that ECT is rarely of value specifically for schizophrenic symptoms, a trial might be warranted if sustained depression dominates the patient's mental state and the risk of suicide continues to be appreciable. It is fortunate that good anesthetic practice can nowadays ensure that the risk of ECT among the elderly is no greater than among younger subjects; radical treatment should not be withheld solely on the grounds of age.

For those less acutely depressed, antidepressant drugs may have a role if the clinician is confident that the patient can be safely supported, whether as an inpatient or an outpatient, for the few weeks that may be required until the drugs have their full effect. A difficulty that sometimes arises is that antidepressants have already been prescribed but then taken in overdose in a parasuicidal act. Some would judge such a sequence as adequate demonstration of inefficacy of the treatment regime and would proceed to ECT. But there may be grounds for deciding otherwise, i.e., from the history of the therapeutic response on earlier occasions (given adequate dosage, etc). If so, and if the antidepressant medication is to continue on an outpatient basis, it is wise to entrust the drugs to a relative who will dispense them to the patient and supervise his routine. Only a small quantity of tablets should be prescribed at a time so that there is no large amount of dangerous substance being kept in the household.

Second, it is important that whatever the details of the specific therapy being pursued the clinician must try to establish a therapeutic relationship with the patient, which is to say that he must provide some form of psychotherapy, however simple. Some general points may be noted.

The psychiatrist himself must have the ability to withstand the anxiety generated by working with suicidal patients. He should never assume role responsibility for such a patient before he has completed his own basic training in psychiatry and has acquired the rudiments of psychotherapeutic skills. If even after this time he finds himself—as he is almost bound to do in most working situations—confronted by a suicidal hazard which he finds oppressive, he would be wise to seek consultation from his colleagues, if only to share with them his preoccupations and to enlist their comment about the course of therapy. But complete freedom from anxiety will never be attained, and indeed it seems that for some patients a measure of anxiety on the part of the therapist is an essential component of successful therapy. This is not necessarily because of hostility; a patient with profound self-doubts may only recognize the countervailing concern for his well-being which he so desperately needs if it is manifest as anxiety on the part of his therapist.

The patient should be helped to focus his thoughts again on the possibility of a future. This can be promoted if small steps can be taken in the course of every encounter to affirm the reality of the days or weeks to follow. For example, even so trivial a matter as engaging the patient in a discussion about the optimal time of the next meeting already begins to draw him into considering the reality of a future.

The therapist should never allow himself to be involved in philosophical debates as to whether life is worth living. Life is sustained not by reasons but by appetites, and questions posed by patients in philosophical terms should be responded to by pursuit of the underlying feeling-tone and its clarification. This strategy does not in any sense imply that "rational" therapies are irrelevant. For example, Beck (28) has developed a system of psychotherapy for depressed patients aimed at rectifying cognitive distortions. Essentially the method focuses on the way in which the depressed patient misperceives his environment and then confounds his problem by applying a faulty logic. Exploration of such issues may be very helpful to the suicidal patient if he is well enough to cooperate.

The choice of psychotherapeutic setting must be considered. Most clinicians would opt for individual rather than group psychotherapy, but the problem does occasionally arise as, for example, with inpatient therapies conducted in wards where psychotherapy is the predominant treatment activity. When a suicidal patient joins such a group the other members often prove to be very protective, refraining from too-detailed questions and providing sensitive support. But the process needs to be watched very carefully. A fragile group can be panicked by a patient preoccupied with suicidal fantasies, and such a patient will then need to be protected by the therapist from the retaliatory activities of the other group members. On balance, most clinicians would probably prefer to avoid exposing suicidal patients to the hazard.

Nothing that has been said should imply that the treatment of the suicidal patient is a matter solely for the therapist and patient as an isolated pair. It was implicit in the above discussion of ward management that in modern psychiatric practice the physician is only one of a team. The same is true, to a varying degree, of ambulatory treatment. The nurse, the psychologist, and above all the social worker may all have an essential contribution to make, though the patient must be quite clear that his primary time of communication is with one clearly identified individual.

SUPPORT AND FOLLOW-UP

The point has been made that the resolution of a depressive phase is sometimes a protracted matter. No problem arises in those rather uncommon cases where a depressive period terminates in a hypomanic swing, however mild. Much more usual is a slow return to normality, which takes longer than either the patient or the therapist realizes at the time, so great is their mutual relief at having passed through the worst part of the depression. It has also been noted that premature termination of contact may be associated with suicide even if there has already been substantial amelioration of mood. The conclusions to be drawn are that termination of therapy should occur by spacing of contacts rather than abruptly, and it should be fully discussed with both the patient and his future "caretakers."

The possibility is sometimes raised of establishing special aftercare services for patients who at some point have been at high risk for suicide even if the acute phase of their disorder has passed. The great drawback of such projects is that in order to identify the majority of future suicides, comparatively broad criteria have to be used. These will bring into the group for future surveillance large numbers of false positives. The logistics of the exercise then become quite impossible. Rosen (29) provided an arithmetical analysis of the problem which has not been challenged (see also review by Kreitman (30)). Moreover, long range prediction becomes increasingly difficult as unforseen events will occur in unforseeable circumstances; the future deaths of family members are an obvious case in point. At the moment the general psychiatric services provide the only realistic mechanism for prophylaxis, and this in turn implies selectivity for longer term follow-up.

An alternative is to make use of comprehensive "at risk" registers maintained by the better organized primary care services. Typically these will include such groups as, for example, those aged over 65 who are living alone, and will ensure that individuals on the register are visited periodically to check on their social, physical, and psychological well-being.

THE AFTERMATH OF SUICIDE

Many potential suicides can be detected by the alert clinician, and perhaps due to his efforts, at least in part, the majority of these will not die. But some will, and the question will then arise as to whether the clinician's responsibilities have ended at that point. There are two further functions which he may appropriately be called on to discharge, one in the immediate aftermath of the death and the second at longer range.

First is the task of dealing with the impact of the suicide upon his colleagues, himself, and perhaps his organization if he is working within a service framework as will generally be the case. The range of people affected may be widespread, including many nonprofessional counselors, crisis intervention staff, psychologists, nurses, psychiatric trainees, and so forth. The immediate impact of a suicidal death can be highly disturbing. Indeed there are reasons why this is so. It has been shown by Andress and Corey (31) that approximately one in four suicides occurs in the presence of another person or while the suicide victim was speaking to someone else by telephone. This proportion refers to a nonhospitalized series, but it serves to make the point that many, perhaps the majority, of suicides occur within an interpersonal context. One of the determinants of the act, in other words, may be precisely to induce feelings of remorse in the people with whom the suicide is involved. (Indeed an argument could be elaborated that suicide always involves a real or actual manipulation of interpersonal relationships, and that far from being a trivial matter, "manipulation" is something which an individual may seek to achieve at the cost of his life.)

Be that as it may, a suicide occurring in, for example, an inpatient setting will not commonly generate great distress among the caring staff. It is good practice always to convene a meeting of the appropriate personnel as soon as possible and to review the events which have led up to it. The details should be systematically covered in a standardized order, drawing on as many sources of information as are available. Particular attention should be paid to the clues which were spotted, if any, as pointers to a future suicide. The original plan of management should be reviewed in an attempt to resolve two rather different issues. The first is whether the various decisions that were made were correct given the information available, whether further data should have been sought at the relevant time, and so forth. The second question is whether the plans that were made were in fact adequately implemented, whether deficiencies in liaison occurred, and whether therapeutic procedures were defective in some way. The conclusions drawn should be directed to the improved management of future patients.

But it would be naive to assume that such a review has nothing but an educational role. Staff members may themselves feel guilty, angry, or anxious about their own part in the events leading up to the death and may tend to blame either themselves or others, appropriately on inappropriately, for real or imagined shortcomings. An important role for the leader of the therapeutic team is to handle such reactions sensitively and to demonstrate by his own example that anxieties can be controlled and indeed harnessed constructively.

This touches on the important question of how the physician should handle his own emotional responses. Though the principles may be the same as those he would employ in supporting his colleagues, they are, of course, more difficult to apply in his own case. It has to be accepted that in the present stage of knowledge it is not always possible to avoid a suicidal outcome. Some deaths of this kind are indeed unpredictable, while others, though perhaps foreseeable, cannot be forestalled despite the most devoted attention. (The latter point is, of course, even more true in general medicine than in psychiatry.) It is also important for the physician to realize that if he is to be effective he must be able to tolerate the loss of a patient. To say this is not to be callous but to recognize that a psychiatrist who collapses in panic in the face of a possible or real suicidal death is of no use to a frightened patient. It will be evident then that a fine balance is required between the physician's compassion, on the one hand, and his ability to withstand his patient's despair, up to and including the point of death, on the other.

The patient's own family is also very likely to be profoundly affected by the suicide. The points to be observed here are much as have already been indicated. A family may be much helped by not only a review of the events around the death, but also by being allowed to ventilate their grief or resentment toward both the deceased patient and toward his mentors, much as would be the case with any other form of bereavement counseling. However, a one-and-for-all encounter of this kind may not be adequate, and the offer of support over a reasonable period of time is sometimes welcomed. It is important also to be particularly careful not to assume that the response of the relatives follows any particular pattern. All kinds of reactions may occur. Most often these are indeed of grieving for the death, but in addition there may be considerable hostility toward the deceased for the reasons already mentioned. Other families again appear to be totally indifferent, or may feel guilty not at their possible contribution to the suicide itself but at their relief at the departure of a family member who may have long been a burden to them, as, for example, a patient with chronic alcohol problems.

All of these steps refer to the period immediately following a suicide. An important longer range activity is the periodic review of suicides formerly known to the doctor or to the service of which he is part but no longer in active care. Much here will depend upon the local organization, but in a standard service operating within a defined community it will usually be possible to arrange by consultation with the local coroner or medical examiner for periodic notifications to be received of all suicides occurring within the area. These names may then be checked against the records of the service, and former cases may be identified. Of course, other ex-patient suicides may have moved out of the area, but the importance of the exercise is clinical rather than epidemiological. Such deaths may be reviewed at, say, annual intervals, drawing on all available evidence. They are best undertaken collectively with several therapeutic teams pooling their expertise. Again the main purpose of the exercise is to learn how clinical practice and service organizations might be improved. But there is a further gain. Unlike reviews held shortly after a death, anxiety is likely to be minimal if only because of the lapse of time and the accumulation of intercurrent events. It is thus less difficult for the participants to discuss matters with the appropriate calmness. By being held regularly such meetings may help to enhance an awareness that suicide can be discussed within a rational framework, that it is part of the natural world, and that as with any other form of death it is one of the hazards of life itself.

References

1. Durkheim E: *Suicide: A Study in Sociology* (translated by Spaulding J, Simpson G). New York, Free Press, 1951.
2. Pokorny AD: A follow-up study of 618 suicidal patients. *Am J Psychiatry* 122;1109–1116, 1966.

3. Guze SB, Robins E: Suicide and primary affective disorders. *Br J Psychiatry* 177:437–438, 1970.
4. Rorsman B: Suicide among Swedish psychiatric patients. *Soc Psychiatry* 8:140–144, 1973.
5. Robins E, Murphy GE, Wilkinson RH, Gassner S, Kayes J: Some clinical considerations in the prevention of suicide based on a study of 134 successful suicides. *Am J Public Health* 49:888–899, 1959.
6. Dorpat TL, Ripley HG: A study of suicide in the Seattle area. *Compr Psychiatry* 1:349–359, 1960.
7. Barraclough B, Bunch B, Nelson B, Sainsbury P: A hundred cases of suicide: clinical aspects. *Br J Psychiatry* 125:355–373, 1974.
8. Chynoweth R, Tonge JI, Armstrong J: Suicide in Brisbane—a retrospective psychosocial study. *Aust NZ J Psychiatry* 14:37–45, 1980.
9. Seager CP, Flood RA: Suicide in Bristol. *Br J Psychiatry* 111:919–932, 1965.
10. Myers DH, Neal CD: Suicide in psychiatric patients. *Br J Psychiatry* 133:38–44, 1978.
11. Roy A: Risk factors for suicide in psychiatric patients. *Arch Gen Psychiatry* 39:1089–1095, 1982.
12. American Psychiatric Association: *Diagnostic and Statistical Manual of Mental Disorders*, ed 3. Washington, DC, American Psychiatric Association, 1980.
13. Feighner JP, Robins E, Guze SB, Woodruff RA, Winokur G, Munoz R: Diagnostic criteria for use in psychiatric research. *Arch Gen Psychiatry* 26:57–63, 1972.
14. Barraclough BM, Pallis DJ: Depression followed by suicide: a comparison of depressed suicides with living depressives. *Psychol Med* 5:55–61, 1975.
15. Murphy GE, Armstrong JW, Hermele SL, Fischer JR, Clendenin WW: Suicide and alcoholism. *Arch Gen Psychiatry* 36:65–69, 1979.
16. Ovenstone IMK, Kreitman N: Two syndromes of suicide. *Br J Psychiatry* 124:336–345, 1974.
17. Breier A, Astrachan BM: Characterization of schizophrenic patients who commit suicide. *Am J Psychiatry* 141:206–209, 1984.
18. Miles CP: Conditions predisposing to suicide: a review. *J Nerv Ment Dis* 164:231–246, 1977.
19. Paerregaard G: Suicide among attempted suicides: a 10 year follow up. *Suicide* 5:140–144, 1975.
20. Tuckman J, Youngman WF: Identifying suicide risk groups among attempted suicides. *Public Health Rep* 78:763–766, 1963.
21. Tuckman J, Youngman WF: Suicide risk among persons attempting suicide. *Public Health Rep* 78:585–587, 1963.
22. Kreitman N: Age and parasuicide ("attempted suicide"). *Psychol Med* 6:113–121, 1976.
23. Garzotto N, Buglass D, Holding TA, Kreitman N: Aspects of suicide and parasuicide. *Acta Psychiatr Scand* 56:204–214, 1977.
24. Fowler RC, Tsuang MT, Kronfol Z: Communication of suicidal intent and suicide in unipolar depression. *J Affect Dis* 1:219–225, 1979.
25. Beck AT, Kovacs M, Weissman A: Hopelessness and suicidal behavior. *JAMA* 234:1146–1149, 1975.
26. Dyer JAT, Kreitman N: Hopelessness, depression and suicidal intent in parasuicide. *Br J Psychiatry* 144:127–133, 1984.
27. Roy A: Family history of suicide. *Arch Gen Psychiatry* 40:971–974, 1983.
28. Beck AT: *Cognitive Therapy and the Emotional Disorders*. New York. International Universities Press, 1976.
29. Rosen A: Detection of suicidal patients: an example of some limitations in the prediction of infrequent events. *J Consult Psychol* 13:397–403, 1954.
30. Kreitman N: How useful is the prediction of suicide following parasuicide? *Bibl Psychiatr* 162:77, 1982.
31. Andress VR, Corey DM: Survivor-victims: who discovers or witnesses suicide? *Psychol Rep* 42:759–764, 1978.

Index

Page numbers in italics denote figures; those followed by "t" denote tables.

correlation with platelet MAO, 54
in brains of suicide victims, 48, 49t
relationship to suicidal behavior, 54, 55t
5-Hydroxytryptophan 58–59, 61
Hyperparathyroidism, 165
Hypertension, 153, 156t, 163–164
Hypnotics, 175
Hypothalamic-pituitary-thyroid axis, 60–62, 165
Hysteria, 171

Illness, physical, 37
[³H]Imipramine binding, 53, 58
Impact of suicidal death, immediate, 193
Impulsivity, and serotonin, 63–64
Incidence of suicide
changes by sex and age in selected countries, 28t
in alcoholism, 91
Indians, North American, 139
Individual features, 187–188
Influenza, 164
Inimical behavior, 2
Initiation, 2
Inpatient setting, and aftermath of suicide, 193
Intent, suicidal, 176
behavior differences related to, 79t
communication of, 11–12, 129, 132
demographic characteristics, 79t
denial of, 187
estimation of degree in adolescents, 147
seriousness of, 187
Intermediate response to suicide, 14–15
Internal attitude, common, 7–8
Interpersonal act in suicide, common, 11–12, 188
Interpersonal loss, alcoholic suicide and, 92, 94
Ireland
religious affiliation and suicide rates, 25
suicide rates, 20

Kidney, transplant and dialysis, 163
Klinefelter's syndrome, 166
Knowledge of the death potential of act, 2

Lethality
monitoring of, 15
perturbation and, 13–14
Life events
and suicide, 36
schizophrenic suicide and, 103
Lithium, 44, 82, 172
Liver disease, 162
Logic of suicidal person, 9
Long range review, 194

Loss
associated with life events, schizophrenic suicide and, 103
by separation from spouse or parent and alcoholism, 184
interpersonal and alcoholic suicide, 92, 94
of self, 13
of will, 2
Lysergic acid diethylamide (LSD), 47

Magnesium, CSF, 59
Management of suicidal person
disposition and, 188–190
inpatient care, 188–190
outpatient care, 190
general principles, 190–192
intermediate and long range effectiveness, 14–15
stratagems, 15
Manic depression, 54, 114
mood swings and, 188
prevention of suicide and, 131
Manic-depressive psychoses, 77
MAO (*see* Monoamine oxidase)
Marital separation, 92, 93
Marital status, 183
and adolescent suicide, 139
and incidence of suicide in schizophrenia, 99
Mass suicide, 116–118
Means of suicide (*see* Methods and means of suicide)
Mechanism, 10
Media reporting, 144–145
Medical contact, relationship to recency and death of depressive, 81t
Medical treatment, prescribed at time of death, 82t
Melancholia
abnormal DST and, 60
diagnosis and suicidal intent, 167
5-HIAA concentrations, 51
plasma free tryptophan concentrations and, 52
Melatonin, plasma, 59
Mental illness, 132
Methods or means of suicide (*see also* specific method)
and trend in suicide rates in England, 29
by adolescents, 140–141t
in schizophrenia, 101
increased availability and adolescent suicide, 145
reduced availability, 146
3-Methoxy-4-hydroxyphenyl glycol (MHPG), 52, 59–60
Methyldopa, 164
Monitoring of lethality, 15